PERGAMON GENERAL PSYCHOLOGY SERIES

Editors: Arnold P. Goldstein, *Syracuse University*
Leonard Krasner, *SUNY, Stony Brook*

Mental Health Issues and the Urban Poor

PGPS-44

Mental Health Issues
and
the Urban Poor

DOROTHY ALITA EVANS, Ph.D.

Alexandria Community Mental Health Center
Alexandria, Virginia

and

WILLIAM L. CLAIBORN, Ph.D.

University of Maryland
College Park, Maryland

PERGAMON PRESS INC.

New York · Toronto · Oxford · Sydney

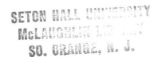

PERGAMON PRESS INC.
Maxwell House, Fairview Park, Elmsford, N.Y. 10523

PERGAMON OF CANADA LTD.
207 Queen's Quay West, Toronto 117, Ontario

PERGAMON PRESS LTD.
Headington Hill Hall, Oxford

PERGAMON PRESS (AUST.) PTY. LTD.
Rushcutters Bay, Sydney, N.S.W.

Library of Congress Cataloging in Publication Data
Main entry under title:

Mental health issues and the urban poor.

(Pergamon general psychology series, 44)
"Contains expanded versions of papers presented at
the Third Annual Symposium on Current Issues in
Community-Clinical Psychology...held at the University
of Maryland, March, 1973."
    Bibliography: p.
    1. Community mental health services--Congresses.
2. Psychotherapy--Congresses. 3. Poverty--
Psychological aspects--Congresses. I. Evans,
Dorothy Alita, ed. II. Claiborn, William L., ed.
III. Symposium on Current Issues in Community-Clinical
Psychology, 3d, University of Maryland, 1973.
[DNLM: 1. Community mental health services--U.S.--
Congresses. 2. Poverty--U.S.--Congresses. 3. Urban
population--U.S.--Congresses. WM30 S995m 1974]
RA790.M363   1974   362.2'2   73-19708
ISBN 0-08-017831-6
ISBN 0-08-017830-8 (pbk.)

Printed in the United States of America

Contents

v

Contributing Authors

Billingsley, Andrew, Ph.D., Vice President for Academic Affairs, Howard University, Washington, D.C.

Dunn, Peter B., M.D., Third Year Psychiatric Resident, Tremont Crisis Center, Bronx State Hospital, Department of Psychiatry, Albert Einstein College of Medicine, New York, New York.

Foley, Henry A., Ph.D., Health Economist, Office of Program Planning and Evaluation, National Institute of Mental Health, Rockville, Maryland.

Goldberg, Carl, Ph.D., Director, Laurel Comprehensive Community Mental Health Center, Prince George's County, Maryland.

Kane, Joyce D., M.S.W., Social Worker, Model Neighborhood Area Comprehensive Community Mental Health Center, Prince George's County, Maryland.

Lerner, Barbara, Ph.D., Consulting Psychologist and Associate Professor, Roosevelt University, Chicago, Illinois.

Ranz, Jules M., M.D., Assistant Director, Tremont Crisis Center, Bronx State Hospital, and Clinical Instructor, Department of Psychiatry, Albert Einstein College of Medicine, New York, New York.

Reiff, Robert, Ph.D., Professor and Director, Center for the Study of Social Intervention, Albert Einstein College of Medicine, New York, New York.

Riessman, Frank, Ph.D., Director, New Human Services Institute, New York, New York.

Schlesinger, Lawrence E., Ph.D., Director of Research, National Children's Rehabilitation Center, Leesburg, Virginia; adjunct staff, National Training Laboratories, Arlington, Virginia.

Shore, Milton F., Ph.D., Clinical Psychologist, Mental Health Study Center, National Institute of Mental Health, Adelphi, Maryland.

Wolpe, Zelda A., Ph.D., Consulting Psychologist, Los Angeles, California.

Preface

THIS BOOK contains expanded versions of papers presented at the Third
Annual Symposium on Current Issues in Community-Clinical Psychology: Mental Health Issues and the Urban Poor, held at the University of
Maryland, March 1973. The sponsors of the Symposium were the Department of Psychology of the University of Maryland and the Maryland
State Department of Health and Mental Hygiene. The conference was
attended by approximately 110 mental health professionals, paraprofessionals, and students in social work, psychology, and psychiatry, as well
as a few poor citizens of urban communities.

The planners of the Symposium aimed to provide, via papers and workshops, a forum in which current mental health theory and technology
were examined for their relevance to the problems in coping faced by
poor people living in urban communities. Such an examination seemed
timely for the following reasons:

1. There is considerable uncertainty about the continued federal support of mental health programs, including those designed to serve the
poor.

2. The quality of life in urban settings continues to deteriorate, as
evidenced in part by the mass exodus of monied people from cities and
given the decline of federally funded Great Society programs for the
poor.

3. The early 1970s seem to be a period of national disillusionment about
how to serve poor people.

The contributions selected for the Symposium and for this book followed a nationwide invitation to professionals and paraprofessionals who work with the poor. Five of the chapters were selected from a pool of papers originally submitted for consideration, plus the invited papers of five leading authorities: Drs. Andrew Billingsley, Barbara Lerner, Robert Reiff, Frank Riessman, and Milton Shore. In addition, to provide organization, continuity, and perspective, the editors contributed introductory and concluding chapters and critical introductions to the other chapters.

Contributions for this book were chosen to represent the most current and in-depth thinking of scholars and practitioners on issues of social value, theory, and practice as they affect the quality of mental health service given to the poor. The book is designed to offer fresh and realistic perspectives to those mental health professionals and new careerists who work with the poor.

The successful culmination of the Symposium and the book reflects the interest and generous cooperation of many people. We especially appreciate the support of Dr. C. J. Bartlett, Chairman, Department of Psychology, University of Maryland; Dr. Forrest B. Tyler, Director, Clinical Training Program, University of Maryland; Dr. Gerry Specter, Mmes. Barbara Henry, Jan Shimerdla, Irma Nicholson, and Mssr. Wayne Brown. The necessary financial support for the Symposium on which this book is based came from registration fees, the Maryland State Department of Health and Mental Hygiene, and the National Institute of Mental Health.

College Park, Maryland   D.E.
                                                                           W.C.

The Editors

Dorothy A. Evans (Ph.D., Southern Illinois University, 1968) is Chief Clinical Psychologist and Director of Research and Evaluation, Alexandria Community Mental Health Center, Alexandria, Virginia. Her primary professional interests are in the delivery of mental health services, professional training of clinical psychologists, mental health consultation, and the development and evaluation of mental health programs for the urban poor. Dr. Evans is a member of several professional associations, has served on the Psychology Training Review Committee of the National Institute of Mental Health, and has been a Visiting Psychologist for the American Psychological Association. Her published works are in the areas of personality correlates of social action, and mental health consultation to antipoverty programs.

William L. Claiborn (Ph.D., Syracuse University, 1968) trained as a clinical psychologist, has professional interests in community and public psychology, especially administration of mental health delivery systems, program evaluation and effects of social institutions. He has published papers in a number of journals and is the co-editor of two volumes: *School Intervention* and *Crisis Intervention*.

Part I

Introduction

CHAPTER 1

Trends and Issues

In the mental health fields the decade of the 1960s was highlighted by efforts to increase the availability and helpfulness of mental health services for poor people. So far, the 1970s have been a more refractory period in which previous efforts are being reviewed to determine what the mental health fields can and cannot offer to help solve the causes and problems of living in poverty. The chapters in this book reflect some of the recent activity of the mental health fields in relation to poverty, and in them are offered some perspectives from which one can conceptualize and plan service roles for work with the poor. This introductory chapter highlights recent trends and issues pertaining to mental health and the urban poor.

In 1963 Congress passed the Community Mental Health Act, which was designed to enable communities to give comprehensive mental health services to all their citizens, including the poor. In addition to the centers for treatment provided by the legislation of 1963, in the early 1960s there were a number of publications on how to treat the mental health problems of poor people. For example, there was Riessman *et al.*'s 1964 benchmark publication of *Mental Health of the Poor: New Treatment Approaches for Low Income People.* Furthermore, there were suggestions that we should shift our focus from the deviant individual to deviancies in social institutions and social values as articulated in Duhl's *The Urban Condition: People and Policy in the Metropolis* (1963). A national endorsement of Duhl's theme was offered in the Great Society legislation and its ensuing social programs of the mid-1960s. In the same time period, mental health fields began to declare a commitment to the idea that

3

misuses of social power and social institutions bear some relationship to the personal adjustment problems of individuals. For example, in 1965 the field of "Community Psychology" was born (Bennett *et al.*, 1966). One of its founding principles was that professional psychology has some responsibility in ameliorating social problems that ensnare people in debilitating circumstances.

Following this ten-year period of activity in the issues of mental health of communities, social institutions, and the poor, the emerging picture is that mental health people are beginning to rethink the question of what they have to offer poor people. For example, it is being asserted that the Comprehensive Community Mental Health centers may not provide viable means for redressing grievances of poor people that are rooted in long-standing social ills (Panzetta, 1971). Also, there is the claim that mental health practitioners have been naive, and perhaps presumptuous, in their attempts to wed political action with clinical practice (Shaw and Eagle, 1971).

The early 1970s seem to be a time in which mental health workers are questioning their responsibility and capability to prevent the causes and ameliorate the dire mental health consequences of living in poverty. Earnest stocktaking requires us to recognize that the mental health fields sometimes have failed to use available knowledge about the problems of poor people in developing intervention programs for the poor. Also, the 1961 Joint Commission Report clearly documents the need for services to the poor (Ewalt, 1961). The Comprehensive Community Mental Health (CCMH) centers were created in spirit to meet this need. The American Psychological Association published a position paper cautioning mental health practitioners about the possible pitfalls in the new CCMH centers (Smith and Hobbs, 1966). Still, even in these centers, the emphasis continues to be on providing services for relatively affluent people (Ryan, 1969). We also know that some mental disorders have been linked to problems in our social systems. Some of these problems are racially prejudicial social policies, systematic denial of social rewards to the poor, and failure to offer poor people an appropriate range of available mental health services (e.g., Duhl, 1963; Kovel, 1971; Miller and Mishler, 1959). Despite these linked issues, there is a strong predilection in the mental health fields to concentrate effort on the victims, without much attention to the social system problems (Caplan and Nelson, 1973).

When efforts have been made to apply conventional mental health theory and practice to the social system underpinnings of the problems of poor people, the results have been mixed (Reiff, 1968; Peck and Kaplan,

1969). Even so, there are those who assert and those who offer empirical support to the view that there are mental health concepts and techniques that have real value for ameliorating the psychological problems related to poverty (Bernard, 1965; Lerner, 1972).

What are the factors that have contributed to the uneven, inconsistent results obtained when mental health experts have attempted to serve poor people? One factor seems to have been enthusiastic but unreflective involvement in politically inspired programs for the poor, and only when it has been socially popular to be involved. Reiff (1971) has noted that social scientists have gotten involved in social issues (e.g., issues such as racial and employment discrimination) only when there has been national consensus to do so. It may be that mental health scientists and practitioners have not engaged in the kind of consistent, systematic efforts necessary to clarify what real contributions they can make to solving personal and social problems related to poverty.

In the 1960s the Great Society zeitgeist provided national government approval to be concerned about poverty. Now, in the 1970s, when the national government is withdrawing support from poverty programs, there is evidence that mental health workers are stepping back some from their involvement with the poor. A pertinent question is whether the mental health fields have a real (i.e., nonpolitical, intrinsic) commitment to understand and aid in the correction of personal problems related to poverty.

Perhaps in the 1970s the question of real commitment will be carefully considered by leaders of the health sciences. The continuing withdrawal of federal fiscal support for mental health training and service (Webb, 1973) may force an answer to this question. In this process, several issues need to be clarified and sorted out. For example, the heightened concern for the poor in the mental health fields during the 1960s paralleled the growth of the CCMH centers and the interest in preventive approaches. The CCMH centers have been offered as the appropriate context within which to treat the problems of poor people, and preventive approaches have been offered as the best strategy for tackling the problems of the poor. The validity of these claims can be established only by further study.

Lerner (1972) cautions us that we may seek new ways of dealing with poor people because our prejudices and stereotyped views of the poor interfere with effective application of the mental health skills already available. Lerner (1972) and others before her (e.g., Smith, 1961; Thomas, 1970) have challenged mental health specialists not to dodge the problems of human and social value involved in serving the poor. It is suggested that social scientists and clinical practitioners fail to consider the extent to which they are "victims" of the prevailing negative stereotyped views of poor people, and that this failure may lead to biased and unhelpful theoretical speculations and interventions.

We are now faced with a kind of fourth revolution in mental health—specifically, the New Federalism (Iscoe, 1973; Webb, 1973). This political philosophy is threatening to radically affect models of training, service, and research in the mental health fields. A probable outcome of the New Federalism, at least over the short term, is less money for mental health programs. If tradition is followed, this probably means that the poor will be the first to lose, and will lose the most. This likelihood sharpens the need of mental health workers to carefully consider their commitments to the poor.

The following chapters are organized into Parts, reflecting several areas of concern about mental health and the urban poor. Following this introduction, in Part II are chapters on values, theory, and research. In Part III are chapters concerned with models for mental health action and problems of the urban poor. In Part IV actual training and service programs related to mental health are described. An overview is provided in Part V.

The offerings of this book are diverse. The diversity owes to the fact that our mental health fields have yet to articulate cohering themes and systematic knowledge and skill in regard to the problems of poor people. Chapters were selected for this book to reflect this inchoateness and (1) to provide the reader with some reasoned speculations as to why the mental health fields seem to be groping vis-à-vis the poor (Part II); (2) to give illustrations of currently available, viable models for service delivery and program planning (Part III); and (3) to provide examples of training and service efforts that have been tried and that seem to be effective (Part IV).

REFERENCES

Bennett, C., Anderson, L., Cooper, S., Hassol, L., Klein, D. C., and Rosenblum, G. (Eds.). *Community Psychology: A report of the Boston Conference on the education of psychologists for community mental health.* Boston: Boston University Press, 1966.

Bernard, V. Some principles of dynamic psychiatry in relation to poverty. *American Journal of Psychiatry*, 1965, **122**(3), 254–267.

Caplan, N. and Nelson, S. On being useful: The nature and consequences of psychological research on social problems. *American Psychologist*, 1973, **28**(3), 199–211.

Duhl, L. (Ed.). *The urban condition: People and policy in the metropolis.* New York: Basic Books, 1963.

Ewalt, J. *Action for mental health.* New York: Basic Books, 1961.

Iscoe, I. The new federalism. *APA Division 27 Newsletter,* 1973, **6**(3), 1.

Kovel, J. *White racism: A psychohistory.* New York: Vintage Books, 1971.

Lerner, B. *Therapy in the ghetto: Political impotence and personal disintegration.* Baltimore: The Johns Hopkins University Press, 1972.

Miller, S. M. and Mishler, E. Social class, mental illness and American psychiatry: An expository review. *Millbank Memorial Fund Quarterly,* 1959, **37**(2), 174–199.

Panzetta, A. *Community mental health: Myth and reality.* Philadelphia: Lea and Febiger, 1971.

Peck, H. and Kaplan, S. A mental health program for an urban multiservice center. In M. Shore and F. Mannino (Eds.), *Mental Health and the Community.* New York: Behavioral Publications, 1969.

Reiff, R. The need for a body of knowledge in community psychology. *American Psychologist,* 1968, **23**(7), 524–531.

Reiff, R. Community psychology and public policy. In G. Rosenblum (Ed.), *Issues in community psychology and preventive mental health.* New York: Behavioral Publications, 1971.

Riessman, F., Cohen, J., and Pearl, A. *Mental health of the poor: New treatment approaches for low income people.* New York: The Free Press, 1964.

Ryan, W. *Distress in the city.* Cleveland: Case Western Reserve University Press, 1969.

Shaw, R. and Eagle, C. Programmed failure: The Lincoln Hospital story. *Community Mental Health Journal,* 1971, 7(4), 255–263.

Smith, M. "Mental Health" reconsidered: A special case of the problem of values in psychology. *American Psychologist,* 1961, **16**, 299–306.

Smith, M. and Hobbs, N. The community and the community mental health center. *American Psychologist,* 1966, **21**, 499–509.

Thomas, C. Psychologists, psychology and the Black community. In F. Korten *et al.* (Eds.), *Psychology and the problems of society.* Washington, D.C.: American Psychological Association, 1970.

Webb, W. Turning point for psychology support. *APA Monitor,* 1973, **4**(14), 2.

Part II

Values, Theory, and Research

CHAPTER 2

Social Action and Community Mental Health

MOST MENTAL health professionals share the belief that social, economic, and environmental factors make a major, if not overwhelming, contribution to the development of psychopathology among the poor. As a consequence, activities involving the professional, his clinic, and his clients in attempts to ameliorate the pathogenic social forces are often seen as a necessary effective strategy. Reiff reviews the logical argument for social activism in CMH, demonstrating that many mental health workers have confused the distinction between value and logical deduction. Reiff provides a careful analysis of the assumption about the causes of pathology (situational, psychological, social structural, and physiological) and the implications of giving priority to one set of causal factors over another. For example, the practice of traditional psychotherapy has focused on producing changes in the individual or psychological causes of pathology, and it has been this level of intervention that has been clearly supported by tradition and funding of CMH centers. Consequently, professionals enlightened to situational and social structural causes of psychopathology have been forced to seek support in non-mental health organizations or to attempt to change their mental health organization to a political one. This has led to the justification of political operations with a mental health rationale. This rationale, according to Reiff, is often specious or at best self-serving. Ironically, the concentration and education on the causes of psychopathology have not provided the mental health worker with knowledge about what produces mental health or competence. A responsible program of social action requires knowledge that the consequences and the process produce improvement in mental health. Reiff suggests that such knowledge is not readily available.

Confusing a social *movement* organization (working for social change) with a social *service* organization (providing assistance to people in need) may produce conflicts in goals, techniques, and rationale. Often the requirements for membership, commitment, and action differ irreconcilably and the end goals may require conflicting changes at different levels of social structure. What is individually therapeutic may have a negative impact on producing change in social structure. Similarly, efforts at radical reform of the social structure may be, at least at the time, destructive to the mental health of the individual.

Being competent at social structural change requires the ability to analyze social policy, to plan and evaluate strategies, to build and use constituencies, and to develop an organization. Mental health professionals are, by tradition, unschooled in these skills. For Reiff, the appropriate role for the professional in the CMH center includes (1) service delivery, (2) educating the community about the pathogenic nature of social conditions, (3) obtaining community support for mental health programs, and (4) creating a change in the immediate social situation that will help the individual.

Reiff's analysis deserves close attention. Predictable progressive social change will require strategies unencumbered by muddled conceptualizing and self-defeating naive ideologists. This chapter by Reiff may help mental health workers sharpen their focus and increase their effectiveness in reaching either goals of service or of social change.

The Social Responsibility of Community Mental Health Centers

ROBERT REIFF

IN THEIR INITIAL enthusiasm for the concept of community mental health some hailed the movement as a "third revolution," anticipating that it would introduce changes in our social institutions on a scale comparable with those of the industrial revolution. Even the more realistic majority viewed community mental health programs as centers of activity that would not only strengthen services for the mentally ill but might also ameliorate social problems and improve the conditions and quality of urban life. The community mental health movement appeared to offer a vehicle through which mental health professionals could transcend their traditional preoccupation with inner psychological processes and move to more active and direct concern with social forces impinging on the individual.

It was not surprising therefore that many clinicians urged that community mental health centers, which deal primarily with the lower socioeconomic groups, develop programs aimed at restructuring and reforming the social fabric of our society, i.e., by bringing about some change in the social institutions and organizations that they believed contribute toward producing the patients with whom they are involved. The more socially conscious among them attempted to give high priority to the development of a social change agent component in community mental health programs. The target population was to be the poor, those in greatest risk of developing a mental illness.

From the very beginning, there was ambiguity about two perspectives of the community mental health concept—its commitment to service and treatment and its commitment to social change. More than ten years of experience have not resolved that ambiguity. Basically, the community mental health center concept assumed that it was possible for a center to carry out both commitments simultaneously. The ideal community mental health center was one in which there was a significant primary prevention program with a heavy emphasis on social change and an extensive network of service and treatment that would take care of the needs of all of the mentally ill in the center's catchment area.

The Community Mental Health Services Act, as distinct from the concept, provided financial support for facilities for the more seriously mentally ill. It clearly mandated that the highest priority should go to the *population in greatest risk of hospitalization.* It provided funds for rehabilitation and treatment services, but no funds for preventive social change programs.

The effect of the Community Mental Health Services Act was to provide facilities and funds for the most seriously mentally ill among the poor, those with the greatest risk of hospitalization, as the target population with the highest priority. The more socially oriented mental health professionals, who took seriously the mandate of the community mental health centers concept for a heavy emphasis on prevention and who considered *all* the poor—the group in society with the *greatest risk of mental illness*—as the target population, were forced to turn to the poverty programs for support. This resulted in two kinds of community mental health centers: those whose resources were devoted primarily to rendering services to the most seriously mentally ill among the poor and those with major social action components aimed at producing changes in the social fabric of the poor.

The fact that the funding came from poverty programs, and in particular the community action section of the poverty programs, compelled the mental health professional to build a strong social action component into his center's program.

The funding from the poverty programs would not have been forthcoming without the employment of indigenous nonprofessionals. The employment of nonprofessionals with poverty program funds infused the mental health program with the political ideology of the antipoverty movement.

The mental health clinician was caught between two ideologies with different purposes: his mental health service ideology, which was primarily treatment-oriented, and the political activist ideology of the antipoverty movement, which was fundamentally antiprofessional, antitreatment, and highly critical of the mental health ideology.

This clash of ideologies and purposes resulted in several "confrontations" that all but wrecked the programs of some community mental health centers.

The drying up of poverty funds has left the mental health clinician with remnants of nonprofessional programs. Today, with no conceptual framework, no body of knowledge, no expertise, and a sense of disillusionment, the question is poised more poignantly than ever. What *is* the social responsibility of community mental health centers? If one holds on

to the conviction, which most of us do, that social disorganization, poverty, racism, drug abuse, and other social problems are causal or contributing factors in the development of a mental illness, what is the community mental health center's responsibility vis-à-vis these problems? I
shall try to present a conceptual framework that I believe can be helpful
in attempting an answer to this question. I will also pose some questions
without answers at the present time, and I will raise some issues that have
not as yet, to my knowledge, been addressed by the mental health professional in the community mental health center.

Let us start with the various possible classes of causal and contributing
factors in the development of a mental illness. There is, of course, the
class of factors that generally are called "physical." The assumption here
is that biological and/or physiological factors are basically responsible for
mental illness. It is, of course, possible that the evils of society are not
causing mental illness but are caused by it, that the history of man with
violence, oppression, slavery, and genocide is a history of a "sick
species"—a point of view somewhat implicit in Freudian theory. If one
actually takes that point of view, the task of curing the mental illness
would be to change the characteristics of the species, and one would have
to address oneself to such problems as breeding, selection, and special environments rather than to "treating" individuals. But this approach poses
some very difficult political and moral questions. The values of our society make such activities morally reprehensible and politically impossible.
We would be compelled to wait for further fantastic breakthroughs in
genetics. Vis-à-vis social problems, from this point of view, there is little
we can or ought to do because the implicit assumption here is that social
problems are not causative factors in mental illness but are caused by
mentally ill people. Our social responsibility would be limited to the development of political and social programs that are oriented almost completely to the development of habilitative or rehabilitative services.

If physiological—i.e., metabolic, viral, etc.—factors are basically responsible, we are in no better position. Our social responsibility would be
for the development of curative and immunization drug research while
promoting a care delivery system that is ameliorative or rehabilitative.

The second class of factors are those generally referred to as
"psychological." The assumption here is that intrapsychic or interpersonal factors are basically responsible for mental illness. Let me deal first
with the intrapsychic theory vis-à-vis social disorganization. Freudian
theory postulates the intrapsychic condition of man as *cause* and the
social condition of society as *effect*. Culture and society are the product of

man's attempts to provide alternatives to the unbridled gratification of the instincts. Culture and society are the effects of the vicissitudes of instinctual conflict. All of man's culture, for example, results from the repression of infantile sexuality. The pattern of social institutions was set by the guilt arising out of the revolt of the sons against the fathers in the primal horde, and every individual repeats this experience in his personal history. Consequently, the ontological developmental experience of each individual repeats the phylogenetic experience of mankind; the basic nature of social institutions that grew out of that phylogenetic experience are immutable because the same intrapsychic dynamics are ontogenetically repeated in every man. Any attempts to change the fundamental nature of social institutions and social relations are doomed to failure because these are the result of the conflict of instincts repeated in every individual in every generation of man. It was this concept that led Freud to remark that the Russian Revolution was a noble experiment but, because of the instinctual nature of man, it would produce little or no change in the basic nature of social institutions and social relations.

On the other hand, Freud does say that while it is impossible to change the nature of instinctual conflict it is possible to modify the way in which these conflicts are resolved. Thus, the Freudian technique was developed that aims at changing the resolution of instinctual conflict in individuals from a so-called "neurotic" one to a so-called "healthy" one. But herein lies one of the greatest difficulties with Freudian theory. Conceptually, it is postulated that intrapsychic conflicts *common to all men* are responsible for the nature of social organization. The implication is that if one can change the intrapsychic dynamics of all men, i.e., of mankind, changes in the social organization will inevitably follow. On the other hand, technologically, the Freudian system is a technique for changing individual men. It has absolutely nothing to say about how one moves from changing individual men to changing mankind except for a naive utopian hope that if enough individuals are analyzed the world will be a better place in which to live.

This assumption has led to the failure to develop a conceptual framework and technology that will enable us to move from the individual to the social order level. The implication of the theory is that if you change enough individuals you will be able to change society. But there is no technology or concept of how to change *enough* individuals. The question of how you change the intrapsychic dynamics of mankind to change the social order becomes nothing more than the naive assumption that if you change an individual for the better he will work to change society for the better.

Many mental health professionals, particularly those in community mental health wishing to be responsive to the social problems of our day, have tried to find a psychological rationale for social and political positions that they consider to be just. In doing so they have taken mental health concepts out of their contexts and have confused themselves and the public. One example of the attempt to generate a rationale for social and political activity from mental health concepts is the concept of sociotherapy. Implicit in the concept of sociotherapy is the view that as man participates with others in trying to change his social world for the better in the process he himself will change for the better. This concept is supposed to provide the mental health conceptual basis for most of the social action programs associated with community mental health centers. Now, to illustrate the confusion and sloppy thinking rampant in this concept, I want to examine some of its propositions.

Proposition 1:   Increased socialization reduces feelings of isolation and counteracts tendencies to retreat into fantasy. On the face of it, this statement seems patently valid but its validity depends on what is meant by increased socialization. If this is interpreted to mean getting patients involved in rent strikes, social protest movements, etc., then the statement is highly questionable because participation on the part of patients in social movements may not be therapeutic and may even be damaging to both the patient and the social movement. Increased socialization may have a therapeutic effect only if it leads to beneficial and corrective socializing experiences. Advising a patient to join a group can be therapeutic if the therapists can to some degree control the climate of the group so that it will afford the patient the kind of corrective experience he needs and will not tax the patient beyond his fragile tolerances. In most cases such a group would be one that understands that its mission with regard to the individual is therapeutic. But social action and social protest groups do not lend themselves to that degree of control, nor are they in a position to consider the therapeutic needs of individuals in them. Their climate is generally stressful, intense, and inconsiderate of individual needs or psychological tolerances. This proposition then is an extrapolation from a generalization about therapeutic groups where it has some validity to social and political movements where it has little or no validity at all. To advise most patients to participate in social and political movements as a form of therapy is dangerous and professionally irresponsible.

Proposition 2:   Participation in social action programs provides constructive channels for the discharge of aggressive drives. This statement has no validity at all. It stems from the political naivete of the mental health professional who often assumes that if a cause is socially just, any aggression exercise to achieve it is constructive. Professionals seem to be unaware that the struggle for a "just" cause may be as destructive to individual mental health as aggression in the service of a socially destructive cause.

The concept of sociotherapy fails to provide a legitimate psychological rationale for social and political action. At best, it perpetuates naive notions about social and political movements and distorts psychological concepts in a manner confusing to the profession and the public.

These propositions illustrate the futility of attempting to justify on a psychological basis support of programs relating to the more relevant social problems of today. They demonstrate the confusion and false assumptions that result when psychological concepts are automatically translated into social and political ones. Finally, they testify to the impossibility of generating social and political solutions to social problems from mental health concepts.

A third class of factors are those that may be called "situational," i.e., those that have to do with the immediate milieu of a person. They have to do with those limited areas of social life of which he is directly and personally aware—the place to go shopping, his work, his education, his family, the local service agencies, etc., everything within his immediate social milieu. Vis-à-vis social problems, many community mental health centers consider it their responsibility to address themselves to the social setting that is directly open to the individual's personal experience; in fact, this is probably the major thrust of most community mental health centers' community activities.

A fourth class of factors contributing to mental illness are those I call "social structures." These have to do with matters that transcend the immediate milieu of the individual. It has to do with many milieu and their organization into the institutions of society as a whole. These issues have to do with the social structure of society. For example, a man and a woman may experience personal problems in their marriage, the family, and other institutions that bear on them. The social structure issues are certainly influencing, perhaps even causing, the experience of personal problems, but there is little personal awareness of this influence and, even if there were, there is perhaps little that can be done about the social structure in the immediate milieu that is open to change by willful activity. That is not to say that understanding these influences does not help. Understanding of the invisible, out-of-reach social forces contributing to the personal problems of living often help an individual to come to his own terms with these problems, but these are problems that the individual qua individual is not able to do anything about by his willful activity. The individual may join a group or a political party, he may vote a certain way, or he may go on a demonstration. He may do many things whose aim is to alter the social structure.

Given our present state of knowledge and technology, it seems obvious that to base all of our thrust on any one of these four classes of possible factors would be risky and irresponsible. What we can do is to keep all four in mind but to structure them in some order of priority. This is, in fact, the reality of our present mental health service delivery system. Different components of the system have structured services based on different orders of priority of these four classes of etiological possibilities. I would say that conceptually community mental health centers' ordering of priorities would possibly be: situational factors first, psychological factors second, social structure factors third, and physiological factors last. However, as I pointed out at the beginning, some community mental health centers have conceptually placed social structure factors first. Regardless of whether situational or social structure factors are placed first, the conceptual thrust is considered to be social change. It is my personal experience that many community mental health centers are unclear as to what the goals of their social change activities are. Some consider the goal of social change to be *changing individuals to achieve some personal objective*, such as finding and holding a job (rehab, work-for-pay programs, on-the-job training, etc.). Some consider the goal of social change to be changing of individuals to achieve a social goal (e.g., give up racist attitudes). In both of these, the goal of social change activity is to change individuals. Others conceive of the goal of social change as being the change of social structures, institutions, or organizations either to achieve a personal goal or a social goal, such as promoting community-control corps to achieve a redistribution of power in a community. This issue has never been clarified by community mental health centers. Is the goal of their social change activity to produce changes in individuals or to produce changes in social structures—i.e., societal changes—or both? These are important conceptual issues. Social change activities oriented toward individual change are likely to focus on changing sentiments, values, etc. The focus on changing individuals is less threatening to the dominant values of society and to other institutions. To the extent that operative goals are restricted to individual change and are not relevant to control or pressure on other institutions, to political action, or to central societal norms, counter pressures are less likely. It is also well to note that the more one is successful in achieving personal goals the less is one's motivation for achieving social change. If the goal is to achieve both individual and social structural change, then another class of serious issues arises (social movement organizations). Any organized, purposive, and collective attempt of a number of people to structure society and its members, to change individuals or societal institutions and structures, has the characteristics of a social *movement* organization as distinct from a social *service* organization, whose primary goal is rendering a service. A very real question can be raised about the viability of a social movement organization within the framework of a social service organization and institution. There are certain fundamental characteristics of a social movement organization that may be contradictory or antagonistic to the necessary characteristics of a service organization. Such questions as membership requirements and characteristics, goals, strategies, and levels of intervention may create tensions in any organization whose primary social and institutional role is service but which is attempting to engage in social movement organizational activities. For example, with respect to membership requirements, there are two types of social movement organizations: those that are inclusive and those that are exclusive. Inclusive social movement organizations require minimal levels of commitment. Membership is often loose and informal, usually a pledge of general support without specific duties; there is little or no indoctrination period, a minimum of activity from its members is required, and their behavior is not disciplined by imposed organizational goals, policies, and tactics. An exclusive social movement organization demands a high commitment from its members with a high degree of organizational discipline and activity. It makes more extensive demands on the members' energy and time. Any social movement organization may have attributes of both forms of membership, but even the most inclusive organization must have a central cadre with exclusive membership attributes. In the traditional service organization, membership requirements are unique. The client or member is expected to trust and follow the directives of the professional server precisely because he does not have the usual personal, ideological, or political reasons for helping him. This is in direct contradiction to the membership requirements of social movement organizations.

I doubt if there ever has been a community mental health center program oriented toward social change that has purposely thought through and explicitly defined the nature of its membership requirements, the rationale for them, the relationship and viability of these requirements for achieving their social change goals, and the difference between these requirements and those necessary for service. Another crucial issue that has not been clarified is the relationship between the level of interventions for social change and the ultimate level at which change is to be accomplished. It is most often assumed that the level of intervention and the level of desired social change are the same. But it is possible, for example, to intervene at the individual level to achieve organizational change or vice versa. This issue gets at the guts of the question of what is meant by social change.

Does social change mean changing the immediate milieu of a client—i.e., getting a client on a job-training program or finding him a foster home? (Intervening at the milieu or community level to bring about change in an individual client.)

Does social change mean changing the immediate milieu of a class of clients—e.g., developing student self-help tutoring programs to help the slow students? (Intervening at the organizational or system level to bring about change in a particular group.)

Does social change mean changing an organization or agency in the immediate milieu of all the people in the community—e.g., decentralizing the school board? (Intervening at the organizational or system level to bring about change in the system itself.)

Does social change mean changing a social structure or institution for the purpose of changing society itself—e.g., designing an antipoverty program that will eliminate poverty? (Intervening at the social structural level to bring about societal changes.)

These are not all the possibilities but they illustrate the confusion about societal change, for any and all of these have been espoused as the responsibility of community mental health centers.

Given these considerations, what is the justifiable responsibility of community mental health centers with respect to social change? Certainly, changes aimed at modifying the immediate social *situation* of the client are a necessary part of any therapeutic program. Social change activities aimed at involving the community in improving the health and mental health care delivery system must be a responsibility of a community mental health center. And, finally, social change activities directed at producing individual change (attitudes, values, etc.) are justifiable, provided that it is demonstrated that they can be generated from mental health or psychological concepts.

We can, for example, point to the relationship between the crowded conditions of the city, the ghetto, and schizophrenia. Thus, we may support programs aimed at eliminating the ghetto, but we cannot justify our support of such programs on the grounds that, if successful, they will provide the social conditions that will promote "healthier" individuals. The support of social and political programs to eliminate pathogenic social conditions is a legitimate function and responsibility of community mental health centers, but it must be recognized and accepted that we can only generate a negative rationale from mental health concepts. We can legitimately say what we are against and back it up on the basis of our knowledge about mental illness, but we cannot say what we are for and legitimately back it up with knowledge about what produces mental health; thus, we are in a position in which we may *generate* "anti" programs. We can educate the public on the need to eliminate certain pathogenic social conditions, but we are limited to *supporting* on faith, rather than generating, programs that proclaim a positive solution to certain pathogenic social conditions.

Social and political programs to eliminate undesirable social conditions are rarely generated on mental health principles. For the most part, they are usually justified on a social or political rather than a mental health basis. It is only the mental health professional who feels a need to "link" social and political programs to mental health principles, perhaps because he realizes from his experience with mental illness that there must be a link between the social and psychological condition of man. Because he has been brainwashed to believe that if he supports programs that are not generated from psychological concepts, he is not making an objective scientific professional decision, but he is making value judgments that—while they may be appropriate in his citizen role—he considers inappropriate in his professional role.

It is necessary to understand the difference between generating a social and political program and supporting a program. A program is generated when a relationship is established with some body of knowledge or experience that is reasonably or logically related to the nature of the program. Generating a program implies a belief or commitment to the relationship between the program and its ideological roots. But one may support a program either with or without such a commitment to the specific ideological basis on which the program was founded. One may have a different rationale or no rational basis at all and yet legitimately support a program.

The problem is that there is a myth among social scientists and particularly among mental health professionals that it is unprofessional to support a program that cannot be generated from mental health concepts.

Thus, as mental health professionals view it, they can support the struggle for Black power if they can relate it to the psychological concept of a sense of autonomy, but they consider support of it on the basis that it is socially just or politically expedient the function of a citizen and therefore wrong or "unprofessional" for professionals to take such a position.

It becomes apparent that the feeble and muddled attempts by the mental health professional to justify social and political programs relating to poverty, racism, and other social inequities on the basis of mental health concepts are motivated by a desire to support programs that he feels are socially just and by a fear that unless he can generate his support for mental health concepts he will not be acting appropriately as a professional. This brings us to the root of the question posed in the opening paragraph of this paper: What is the responsibility of the community mental health centers in the face of social unrest, poverty, racism, and other social inequities? I have attempted to show that, without question, community mental health centers can generate and support programs that educate the public about the pathogenic nature of these social problems, and they have the responsibility to do so. Community mental health centers also have the responsibility to generate and support programs relating to changes for the improvement of patterns of mental health care and the nature of mental health services. What remains to be discussed is the question: Does the community mental health center have a responsibility to support social and political programs that are considered socially and politically desirable but that cannot be generated from or justified by mental health concepts? Or, to put it another way: Does the mental health profession have a legitimate professional role to play in bringing about social reforms that at the present time cannot be scientifically generated from mental health concepts? If it does, what is that role?

Social change activities whose ultimate goal is to bring about larger societal changes, i.e., changes in the social structure, require:

1. social policy analysis,
2. social program planning and evaluation,
3. constituency building at all levels, and
4. organization and membership.

The first two demand a social science knowledge and skills that go beyond the conceptual framework of the mental health clinician. The second two require the utmost political skills. As I have already noted, it is highly doubtful that the kind of political organization and membership necessary for such political activities can be successfully developed within the framework of a human service organization such as the community mental health center.

The politics of the community mental health center should revolve around programs for the mentally ill, with public educational and lobbying activities for such programs. The primary political activity of a community mental health center should be the development of the community as a constituency for the substantive nature of programs for the mentally ill. The community mental health center can initiate and provide support for activities that increase the client's capacity to exercise his willful activity on the immediate milieu, including developing mechanisms and programs to make it possible for individuals to increase the degree to which the immediate milieu is responsive to their experience and activities. That means:

1. developing a program that adequately meets the constituency's needs,
2. involving community elements as participants in planning and implementation of programs for the mentally ill,
3. educating the community on how to act like a constituency, and
4. educating professionals to accept and utilize the community as a constituency.

The community will probably ask "what's in it for us?" The reply "good service" is not sufficient and will be regarded cynically by the community, so long as there is no accountability or the definition of "good service" is determined by or depends on the whim and the needs of the professional rather than on the community. Some degree of accountability is necessary as a quid pro quo for the community acting as the constituency in the community mental health centers. The degree to which this can be accomplished depends upon the political sophistication of the community, the political resources it can mobilize, and the professional's willingness to function with such accountability.

CHAPTER 3

Victim Blame and Mental Health

BILLINGSLEY NOTES the proclivity of mental health scientists to examine only the contributions sufferers make to their own suffering (Billingsley, 1968). In this paper, the "victim blame" approach is examined in terms of the thesis that much of what we label mental illness in the individual is a mere manifestation of misdirected social values, structures, and practices. It is proffered that many so-called mental illnesses represent psychologically cogent attempts at accommodating social stress.

Billingsley probes possible reasons for what he sees as an unfortunate need on the part of mental health scientists to concentrate on the reasonable accommodations individuals make, especially economically poor people, to societal forces antagonistic to individual growth and development. It is argued that we need to examine closely broad-scale social policy and values as well as individual adjustment patterns. Billingsley suggests that in so doing we will find that mental health concepts and practices are tainted by our nation's overinvestment in the acquisition of social power. Billingsley believes that we fix our theorizing and mental health practices on individuals, particularly the socially most disadvantaged individuals, in order not to examine and thereby risk disruption in those societal structures and practices that nurture our investment in social power.

Billingsley points out that it has become fashionable among mental health specialists to espouse a high priority investment in the development of broad mental health conceptions sensitive to the deleterious effects of particular social institutions and practices (e.g., racism and the quest for social power). We are exhorted to increase our professional

25

candor by translating our "highfalutin" words into careful programmatic effort. Caplan and Nelson (1973) adroitly clarify the urgent need for the kinds of refocusing that Billingsley suggests; specifically, the need to study and to help eliminate the societal underpinnings of personal distress, as well as to continue our inquiry into individual suffering.

REFERENCES

Billingsley, A. *Black families in white America.* Englewood Cliffs, New Jersey: Prentice-Hall, 1968.
Caplan, N. and Nelson, S. On being useful: The nature and consequences of psychological research on social problems. *American Psychologist,* 1973, **28**(3), 199–211.

The Struggle for Mental Health

ANDREW BILLINGSLEY

IN THE FIELD of mental health the questions uppermost in the minds of all of us are these: How can we maintain or recapture our mental health at a time and in a society where all the major forces are arrayed against us? How can we maintain our sense of worth, our sense of balance, our ability to function and to cope with the vicissitudes of life and to exploit to the fullest the opportunities in life in order to contribute toward a more humane society? How can we maintain or recapture our mental health as individuals, as groups, and as a society? Like all other major goals, it is a struggle. It is not easy.

All around us today there are signs that individuals, families, institutions, and communities have lost the struggle for mental health. The problem is serious, is of enormous magnitude, and is growing rapidly every day. Altogether, in 1970 there were nearly a million individuals confined to mental hospitals, almost a million confined to homes for the aged, and over 775,000 confined to other types of institutions.

In these circumstances somebody has made the decision that these individuals cannot cope with society and must be removed from their homes, their families, and their communities. Sometimes the decision is voluntary—the individual has some say about his and her removal. More often, the decision is involuntary, in the sense that somebody else makes the decision that these individuals should be removed from society for their own protection, for their own benefit, for their own welfare, and for the protection, the benefit, and the welfare of the larger society. But the institutionalized populations constitute only the tip of the iceberg. It is only one barometer of the status of emotional and social well-being in our society. It calls our attention to the fact that something is out of kilter, something has gone wrong.

In the southern part of the United States, where the rate of incarceration is highest, there are nearly 1.9 million persons incarcerated in these various types of institutions. In the north-central part of the country there are 1.5 million; in the northeast there are 1.3 million; and in the far west, where there are not many people, only a million are incarcerated in institutions including mental hospitals, homes for the aged, prisons, and other forms of isolation.

Another sign of the tremendous social disequilibrium that we are experiencing may be found in the incidence of geographic mobility. In 1970 nearly 51 million people, or more than a quarter of the total population, resided in a different state from which they were born. In the southern part of the country, where this phenomenon is highest, this represented more than 19 million individuals so relocated; in the north-central region—more than 15 million; in the northeast—nearly 11 million; and in the far west— 5.5 million individuals so relocated. It cannot be suggested that migration in itself is a sign of mental illness on the part of the migrants in any classical definition of that term. We know from the work of demographers and other social scientists that people move for two basic reasons. There is a set of dissatisfactions with where they are—called the push factor— which pushes them out of their homestead, and there is a set of real and imagined opportunities that leads them to relocate in other places—these are the pull factors.

At the same time, however, whatever the basic reasons for such tremendous movement, it is also clear to us that such mass migration represents tremendous social flux and is both a reflection and a source of much of the malaise, the discontent, the lack of a sense of well-being on the part of our large, sprawling, complex population. In this light, then, let us consider the matter of relocation and dislocation in a bit more detail.

Since 1965 alone, among people five years old and over, over 75 million people have moved to a different house, more than 31 million have moved to a different county, and more than 16 million have moved to a different state.

In addition, the tremendous movements into and out of personal relationships, as represented by the marriage, separation, and divorce statistics, constitute still another level of indicators of mass social disequilibrium. We know, of course, that such separations and rearrangements can be both a problem and a solution to a problem, sometimes both for the same people. Yet, they tell us something about the conditions of life and the stresses of life as we struggle for a sense of belonging, a sense of relatedness, and a sense of well-being.

It must be clear by now that when we speak of mental illness we are not speaking of a narrow conception of that term but of the broad social and personal disequilibrium that we experience. And, when we speak of the struggle for mental health, we refer to the efforts we make individually and collectively to find or restore increasing levels of personal and social equilibrium. The struggle for mental health, then, is our effort to adapt to, resist, and take advantage of the strains and stresses of life in order to move toward increasing levels of personal satisfaction and social functioning and toward a sense of personal and social well-being. In this race toward sanity, it often seems that the cards are stacked against us. We seem to have inherited and constructed a society designed to move us all rapidly toward madness, to separate us from our conceptions of ourselves and each other. Mental illness, then, which may be defined as the absence of mental health, is not an abnormal condition. It is a normal response to the conditions of life and society around us.

Children learn this very early in life. In their pioneering and very controversial study of life's stress and mental health in Manhattan a few years ago, Langner and Michael (1963) constructed what they call a childhood mental health index. This was composed of four different sets of responses children made to their inquiries.

They called the first set of responses a childhood neurotic score. Let us observe for a moment the kinds of questions they asked and then let us think, if we will, about our own children and clients and neighbors as we see how these particular researchers established the preconditions of social malfunctioning. They asked the following kinds of questions: As a child, did you fairly often have trouble falling asleep, did you ever have trouble with stuttering or stammering in your speech, did you fairly often have an upset stomach? "Yes" responses to these questions added up to a pattern of childhood neuroticism. Yet each of these, and all of them collectively, are very common and normal features of our everyday life today.

Or consider the second aspect of their index. In this, they inquired into childhood psychosomatic conditions. They wanted to know if children suffered from arthritis, asthma, bladder trouble, hay fever, high blood pressure, skin conditions—all very common, ordinary features of our children's lives today.

Third, they inquired into what they considered a childhood functioning score. In this exercise they wanted to know to what extent the person felt as a child that he was happy only when he was at home, or as a teenager whether he dated girls, or boys, more or less often than others in his age and peer group. Further, they wanted to know whether as a child he liked or disliked school. Observe with me the likely responses in our contemporary, social situation.

Finally, Langner and Michael inquired into what they called childhood fears. They wanted to know if, as a child, these subjects were afraid of strangers, thunderstorms, being left alone, high places, large animals, being laughed at by other children, family quarrels, and getting bawled out. In this study these childhood experiences, feelings, and attitudes added up to a pattern of mental health or ill health, depending on how the respondents answered the questions. Thus, while mental health is a goal highly to be desired and sought after, the absence of it is not a sign of deviance or abnormality, but is a normal part of our everyday lives.

A few years ago Jerry Gurin and his associates at the University of Michigan did a national study called *Americans View Their Mental Health*. It was a study designed "to investigate the level at which people are living with themselves—their fears and anxieties, their strengths and resources, the problems they face and the ways they cope with them." In Part I of their findings, they described some of life's satisfactions and dissatisfactions, tensions and concerns, and sources of happiness and strength that were experienced by a representative sample of the adult population of the United States at that time. They examined the sources of happiness and unhappiness in the general population around 1960. They discovered that economic and material considerations constituted both a chief source of happiness in the population and a chief source of unhappiness. They also found, however, that the second major source of both happiness and unhappiness was associated with marriage and children and other aspects of family living. A number of other studies have shown the tremendous interaction among these three variables— economic well-being or strivings, childhood and family life, and satisfaction or distress.

When these scholars zeroed in particularly on the sources of worry among the American people, they found that 41% worried about economic and material conditions, 18% worried about their families' health, 15% worried about their children, and 11% worried about community, national, or world problems. When the respondents were asked how often they worried about these various things, over 40% indicated that they worried all the time. Furthermore, 20% of this national sample felt that they had at sometime experienced a feeling of impending nervous breakdown and another 23% indicated that they had severe personal problems that required professional help. These researchers were particularly intrigued with the fact that more than half of these people who felt impending nervous breakdowns felt no need or use for professional help. The point we are making is that anxiety is a structured feature of American society experienced by a large number of people. It starts very early in life and persists into old age.

The recent findings of the Joint Commission on Mental Health of

Children represent a milestone in national analysis of and prescription for the problem and, indeed, the struggle for mental health among children and families as well (*Report of the Joint Commission on Mental Health of Children*, 1973). More than 13 national, professional associations joined together in forming the board of directors for that massive study and set of recommendations. It was a report to the Congress. In authorizing the establishment of this Joint Commission, the Congress declared as follows:

> This nation, the richest of all world powers, has no unified national commitment to its children and youth. The claim that we are a child-centered society, that we look to our young as tomorrow's leaders is a myth. Our words are made meaningless by our actions, by our lack of national community and personal investment in maintaining the healthy development of our young, by the miniscule amount of economic resources spent in developing our young, by our tendency to rely on a proliferation of simple, one factor, short-term and inexpensive remedies and services .... This nation, which looks to the family to nurture its young gives no real help with child rearing until a child is badly disturbed or disruptive to the community. The discontent, apathy and violence today are a warning that society has not assumed its responsibility to insure an environment which will provide optimum care for its children. The family cannot be allowed to withstand alone the enormous pressures of an increasing technological world. Within the community, some mechanism must be created which will assume the responsibility for assuring the necessary supports for the child and the family .... This nation, highly sophisticated and knowledgeable about mental health and child development, continues its planning and programming largely around the concept of *treating* rather than preventing mental illness. But no agency has the task and responsibility for assuring that treatment is, in fact, received by those who need it.

In submitting its final report, the Commission gave concrete evidence of the sad state of our mental health programs to the Congress. The Commission stated:

> We join forces with those who propose a broader, but more meaningful concept of mental health, one which is based on the developmental view with prevention and optimum mental health as a major goal. We contend that the mentally healthy life is one in which self-direction and satisfying interdependent relationships prevail, one in which there is meaning, purpose and opportunity. We believe that lives that are uprooted, thwarted and denied the growth of their inherent capacities are mentally unhealthy, as are those determined by rigidity, conformity, deprivation, impulsivity and hostility. Unfulfilled lives cost us twice—once in the loss of human resources, in the apathetic, unhappy, frustrated and violent souls in our midst, and, again, in the loss of productivity to our society and the economic cost of dependency.

The Commission concluded:

> If we are to optimize the mental health of our young people, we must develop a national commitment, philosophy and programs designed to guarantee children from a very

early age the following basic rights. First, the right to be wanted; second, the right to be born healthy; third, the right to live in a healthy environment; fourth, the right to satisfaction of basic human needs; fifth, the right to continuous, loving care; sixth, the right to acquire the intellectual and emotional skills necessary to achieve individual aspirations and to cope effectively in our society. And, finally, the right to receive care and treatment through facilities which are appropriate to their needs and which keep them as closely as possible within their normal social settings.

It is perhaps particularly appropriate for us to reflect that since 1959 we have as a society made some halting steps in the direction to which the Commission pointed and to which the 1970 White House Conference on Children also subscribed. But candor requires us to observe also that currently the nation seems to be hell-bent on taking a giant step backward from this commitment to the well-being of our children (e.g., the threat of imminent and very sharp reductions in federal monies for social and health-care programs). As a consequence, the struggle for mental health in 1973 takes on new and ominous dimensions.

As a consequence of the strains and stresses in our society, personal and social disintegration are on the increase. The rate of suicide goes up, drug addiction runs rampant in our communities, and young and old people drop out—from life, from school, from family, from selves; large numbers become incarcerated in institutions, and social malaise seems to grow by leaps and bounds. At the very height of all these developments, our national, state, and sometimes even our local government seem to desert us. We who are engaged in the professions of health, education, and human services, who know the value of concerted, collective social solutions to collective social problems, are faced with new challenges, the likes of which we have not faced for a long time in this country.

First, we are challenged to reexamine our own conceptions of mental health. It is one thing to sit in an audience or a workshop and agree or disagree when someone says that we need a broad conception of mental health. It is yet another to return to our own offices and continue practicing and foisting off on our clients, students, neighbors, and friends narrow, rigid, professional, technical approaches that we have inherited from our teachers and their teachers and that help us to become increasingly expert, perhaps increasingly well-off, and at the same time increasingly less useful to the community. We must move, I suggest, beyond the narrow limitations of our specialties, not only in order to be more useful to the community but in order to survive as professionals.

Second, we must critically reexamine our own pet theories, pet projects, and pet programs for their dysfunctions as well as their functions and seek to bring them in line with the real needs of the people rather than keep them consistent with our own theories and preconditions.

Third, we must apply ourselves vigorously as professionals to an analysis of the broad-scale social policies that affect all aspects of our lives, not only those that are specifically earmarked as mental health. In analyzing these policies, we must come to see the interrelatedness of what happens in industry, agriculture, and government with the mental health of our population. But surely analysis is not enough. We must find new ways to assist our government in taking a leadership role to insure that the total institutional fabric of the nation will be devoted to the total well-being of our total population.

In his book, *The Two Worlds of Childhood*, Bronfenbrenner (1970) challenges us as professionals to move from social science to social action without abandoning the insights that come from careful study and analysis. He reminds us of a few things we all know but need to be aware of as we seek to move our society toward a sane society.

Bronfenbrenner writes:

> We now consider how the principles we have derived from research can be applied within the framework of the major American institutions involved in the process of socialization. Clearly, the institution which stands at the core of the process in our own culture is the family. And it is the withdrawal of the family from its child rearing functions that we have identified as a major factor threatening the breakdown of the socialization process in America.

He calls for new patterns of family involvement. He refers specifically to the engagement of parents and older children in new and more mutually rewarding patterns of interactions with younger children in the family. There is a great deal of age segregation, and he calls on us to reverse this tendency.

Calling on some of his own insights from the early days of Head Start, he recommends demonstration programs in school and nonschool programs starting at a very early age. He observes:

> Particularly valuable in this connection are activities that involve and require more than one person in patterns of interaction with the child. That is, not just the teacher and/or the mother, but also other adults and older children, including father, grandmother, brother, sister, and next-door neighbor.

Second, he urges the involvement of parents and neighbors directly in the affairs of the school. For surely, he says, "The most needed innovation in the American classroom today is the involvement of pupils in responsible tasks on behalf of others within the classroom, the school, the neighborhood, and the community." He informs us:

> If the school as a total community becomes visibly involved in activities focused on the child and his needs, if older children, school organizations, other teachers, school administrators, P.T.A.'s—if all these persons and groups in some way participate in the programs and publicly support those most actively engaged in the effort, the reinforcing effect increases by geometric proportions.

But the family and the school are not alone in this effort to increase our sense of belonging and competence. The neighborhood still plays an important role in this process.

He recognizes, as many of us do, that the neighborhood peer group, particularly "the adults and older children who are looked up to and admired by the young, probably stand second only to parents in terms of their power to influence a child's behavior."

He urges educational institutions and professionals of all types to try to exploit and utilize, rather than ignore or go to war with, these peer influences on the young.

Finally, it is in the realm of the larger society outside the neighborhood and community where major reforms are needed to move us toward a sane society. Yet, he would emphasize for us what he calls local initiative and concern.

> We believe that this is the place to start, that is where the children are. For only a hard look at the world in which they live—a world which we adults have created for them in large part by default—can convince us of the urgency of their plight and the consequences of our inaction.

Bronfenbrenner states:

> In summary, it is our view that the phenomenon of segregation by age, and its consequences for human behavior and development, pose problems of the greatest magnitude for the western world in general, and for American society in particular. As we read the evidence, both from our own research and that of others, we cannot escape the conclusion that if the current trend persists, if the institutions of our society continue to remove parents, other adults and older youths from active participation in the lives of children, and if the resulting vacuum is filled by the age-segregated peer group, we can anticipate increased alienation, indifference, antagonism, and violence on the part of the younger generation in all segments of our society—middle-class children as well as the disadvantaged.

So the struggle for mental health, our efforts to find a sense of personal worth, a sense of belonging, a sense of collective well-being, must be waged on the personal level, in the family, in the neighborhood, and in the

Extracts on this and preceding page are from *Two Worlds of Childhood: U.S. and U.S.S.R.* By Urie Bronfenbrenner, © 1970 by Russell Sage Foundation, New York.

larger society. At each of these levels the mental health professions represented can play a crucial role.

In his new book, *Beyond Black and White*, Comer (1972) has reminded us that:

> We live in a society that makes trust and respect difficult. Our social system produces too much uncertainty, fear, and anxiety. This is due largely to the fact that America has a defect in its executive or leadership structure and in its ethical or moral structure, similar to ego and super ego defects or weaknesses in an individual. In fact, the behavior of too much of the leadership group resembles neurotic patterns in individuals—fleeing from responsibility, failing to face up to reality, self-destructiveness.

The struggle for mental health, then, must be waged at the highest level of our society. As Frederick Douglass reminded us a long time ago, it will not be easy, for "power concedes nothing without a struggle. It never has and it never will (Foner, 1950)."

REFERENCES

Bronfenbrenner, U. *Two worlds of childhood: U.S. and U.S.S.R.* New York: Russell Sage Foundation, 1970.

Comer, J. P. *Beyond Black and White.* New York: Quadrangle Books, 1972.

Foner, P. S. (Ed.). *The life and writings of Frederick Douglass.* New York: International Publishers, 1950.

Gurin, G., Veroff, J., and Feld, S. *Americans view their mental health.* New York: Basic Books, 1960.

Langner, T. and Michael, S. T. *Life, stress and mental health.* New York: Macmillan, 1963.

Report of the Joint Commission on Mental Health of Children. New York: Harper & Row, 1973.

CHAPTER 4

Consumer Sensitive Program Planning and Evaluation

FRANK RIESSMAN, well known for being at the forefront of the development of new social services and the full utilization of new forms of manpower, presents some reflections on the current "service consciousness." The coalescing of many factors has led to increasing pressures on social service workers to document their value to the poor and to stand the test of public or peer scrutiny. The new social service roles utilizing paraprofessionals and providing new careers have been carefully developed by mental health professionals or have sprouted indigenously. In most cases the effectiveness of these services is neither defined nor measured. These services are supported instead because they fill a popularly felt need.

Riessman reminds us that it is difficult to find relevant and sharply targeted assessment devices that permit unbiased evaluation without disturbing the ongoing process. His call, often sounded before, is for a multivariate attack on assessment in an effort to develop divergent and discriminant validity. He argues for extending evaluation to the long term and for the examination of both the manifest and latent goals of the program. For Riessman, manifest or stated program goals typically reflect only a portion of the informal expectation for a program and neglect the role that program serves within the zeitgeist. It is shortsighted to judge a program solely by its direct specific achievements while neglecting the program's impact on a community's beliefs and morale. The "psychology" of a program may be far more important than its real achievements. Finally, Riessman proposes the matching of evaluation procedures to the program being evaluated—something that is nearly obvious but seems to get lost in practice.

For Riessman, the flourishing of new professions, new careers, and paraprofessions reflects a basic shift in the organization of service delivery, not in the content of the service. As the open classroom is seen as an effective way to impart the same "scholarship," the paraprofessional mental health worker may be a more effective agent in the therapeutic process. In order to develop improved service delivery, the goals to be achieved must be clearly specified and the programs developed toward that goal. "Goal keying" should determine the organization of the service, the form of the training program, and the choice of the service agent. In an obvious example, working with a Spanish-speaking client, Riessman suggests that a bilingual paraprofessional would be a more appropriate service delivery agent than his more highly trained professional supervisor. The concept of matching service delivery schemes to the particular attributes of the consumer preclude the development of grand generalizations about the most desirable means to deliver service and require that individual study be given to the development of models for mental health service to the poor.

The paraprofessional and professional, therefore, should coexist within the same agency, performing complementary functions uniquely suited to their respective training and attributes. While paraprofessionals should be trained to provide specific service, it is illusory to presume that their training makes them competent to take on all the roles of the professional. For Riessman, then, the professional should retain supervisory responsibility reflecting his broader knowledge. The confusion of roles experienced by the paraprofessional results from a lack of planning in training for specific roles and in guild jealousies that serve to keep new career ladders closed or poor imitations of the professional career opportunities. Riessman believes that lateral transfer of paraprofessional to professional role should be permitted when the paraprofessional develops the skills and knowledge appropriate to the role.

Many changes can be expected in the continuing shift in this country from capital intensive to labor intensive service business. The burgeoning service careers will need organizations to fight for and protect their rights while, at the same time, consumers will begin to take a more direct role in the determination of the type and nature of service provided. Citizen consumers will appear on boards of directors, advisory committees, and evaluation teams. Radical forms of service meeting the needs of the consumer (see Ranz and Dunn, Chapter 9) will make obsolete much in the traditional "professional" service models. Accountability at all levels of service will become increasingly necessary and can best be met by specifying goals of training and service and by developing service delivery strategies that permit effective evaluation. The pressures on fundings for mental health services to the poor can be met with a concerned effort from consumers and service providers.

Whatever the state of affairs, it is important not to use explanations as apologia for inaction.

Service Effectiveness and the Problem of Evaluation

FRANK RIESSMAN

BEGINNING WITH the Black and youth movements of the 1960s and continuing with the women's movement and the taxpayers' revolt of the 1970s, the public services in our society have been under powerful attack. They are variously portrayed as inhumane, ineffective, insensitive to the consumer, unaccountable, not relevant, and lacking in vitality. A rapid rise of what might be called "service consciousness" has taken place; services are carefully scrutinized and evaluated by the user, the community, the public, not merely by the professional and his peers, or the agencies and their executives.* The days of professional and agency autonomy may be numbered; while "peer review" is an important aspect of accountability, it is clearly insufficient in the eyes of the consuming public.

In the 1960s the questions raised by Blacks regarding services led to demands for community control, the employment of neighborhood residents, new forms of work-study, and an open enrollment that hopefully might provide workers who were more effective and thereby produce service work that was more relevant. Youth also were very much concerned with the lack of relevance and vitality of the services they were receiving, such as education, and the services they were preparing to offer, such as medicine and law. Together with small but vocal groups of professionals, students began to develop various forms of alternative institutions, such as people's health centers, half-way houses, hot lines, etc. In the 1970s women added their voices with particular concern for the ways in which various services discriminated against women. They were particularly critical of the health and mental health institutions, and have countered with feminine counselors, "vaginal politics," and the like.

Perhaps the very last to add its voice has been the average middle-class taxpayer, who is complaining about paying increasingly higher taxes for services that don't appear to serve. Arguing that they don't want to hire

*Increasingly there is developing also the idea of services as rights. Long true with regard to elementary and secondary education, the scope of these rights to services has expanded in one degree or another to include higher education, health care, legal services, and rights of the handicapped and mentally ill.

41

more teachers when children don't learn better, these citizens have won the support of an administration that is committed to the cutback of human services for a great variety of reasons, not least of which is the service ethos—an ethos that is also unattractive to most of these same taxpayers. With such an array of opposition, together with the research ranging from Jensen and Jencks to Illich, it is no wonder that the services are on the defensive, that their efficacy as well as their humanity are being deeply questioned.

Thus, there seems to be little question that there is a real need for examining the human services in order to improve their productivity and effectiveness both for strategic and tactical reasons. On principled grounds, it appears essential that the services "serve"; moreover, if they are to expand in our society, they will require the support of a wide array of forces.

While the demand for increased accountability and effectiveness of services has become very prominent, the means for achieving such objectives are not so readily available. For the most part, the initial impact has been indirect or nonspecific. Thus, community advisory boards have been established on the assumption that such community involvement may make the service giver more responsive to the consumer. Paraprofessionals have been employed with the idea that they would bring a community voice into the service system, thereby affecting agencies and professionals. Voucher systems have been experimented with in order to capture some of the presumed power that the buyer of a service may possess. Decentralization has been applied in neighborhood service centers in order to reduce the distance of the client from the service. Competency- or performance-based certification has been advocated in order to identify more closely what the practitioner is able to do. New methods of analyses of the work (e.g., job or functional task analysis) are designed to demystify the work that is done and to bring it under greater scrutiny and control. Advocates and expediters have been employed to cut through red tape and speed service delivery. Consumers have been used as servers in programs such as Youth Tutoring Youth to increase the consumer dimension of the service. Much more developed training designs have been employed, stressing simulation, in the hope that more pinpointed skills will emerge and thus the service will be improved. And, of course, service modalities such as the open classroom, the community mental health center, and many, many more have been introduced on the grounds that they are more involving of the client or consumer and will therefore produce a better service. The organization of roles (differentiated staffing), both professional and paraprofessional, has been proposed as a major device for increasing effectiveness, and the use of new types of personnel (such as generalists, health advocates, multipurpose family workers and the like) have been proposed to represent clients in a better way.

While in some of these illustrations there have been specific measurements related to the effectiveness of new intervention, for the most part they are "accepted" on face value. They appear to have, on the basis of their logic, a likely effect on improving the service or at least on making it more consumer relevant. But, as we shall see, the two are not necessarily identical.*

In addition to all the various approaches mentioned above, alternative institutions such as free schools, sensitivity groups, and growth centers have attempted to organize the services in a different framework with a new ethos, making them more humane and nonbureaucratic, at least in intention. These services are marked by advocacy or commitment orientation; however, there is little direct evidence regarding their effectiveness. They seem to be accepted for the most part because of what they are *trying* to do and their general philosophy rather than on some specific criteria.

In a sense, their effectiveness is judged because we like some of the values they espouse—e.g., participation and mutual help—and perhaps because they seem to enlist a good number of people, many of whom were turned off in the more traditional help systems. Moreover, these people sometimes report that they are helped and this cannot be entirely cast aside, whatever the limitations of subjective reporting.

THE PROBLEM OF EVALUATION

All of this brings us to the need for a strategy of evaluation directed toward the development and the improvement of the human service systems. The problem of evaluation of human services is enormous, perhaps even more complex than it is in the social sciences in general. Let us look at a few examples. If we use achievement or reading test scores to assess the effectiveness of teachers, we are faced with the problem that the teachers may then "teach to the test." In extreme cases, such as one well-known performance contracting example, they may actually provide

---

*Most of the new approaches are predicated on the assumption that there are a variety of traditional norms, practices, and ways of organizing services that are counterproductive, e.g., professionalism, credentialism, hierarchy, bureaucracy, overspecialization, mystification of the service, making clients dependent, etc.

the tests in advance. If we utilize a measure of the student's self-concept as a way of evaluating some educational intervention, the question naturally arises: "Has his self-concept improved while his cognitive performance remained the same?" If we use the teacher's judgment as to what has been happening to the work of the pupils, this obviously has potential bias as the teacher may want to indicate that he or she is doing a good job, while an outside independent judge may be less capable of assessing what is going on every day or may obtain a restricted performance on the day of his evaluation. On and on go the limitations, whether it be of teacher performance, psychotherapy (e.g., the patient's subjective report of being better may illustrate only his brainwashing by the psychiatrist), or other service fields.

What emerges is a need for an evaluation model that employs multiple indices, each different from the other, each subject to different weaknesses and strengths that may counterbalance the other, but converging toward a similar result or assessment. In the psychological literature this is termed *convergent* and *discriminant validity*, (Campbell and Fiske, 1959). Thus, in the case of a psychotherapeutic intervention, if the patient, his friends, relatives, fellow employees, supervisors, psychiatrists, and perhaps an independent judge agree that he has progressed markedly, we may be more persuaded than if any one of them alone so indicated. If, further, there were some measure such as a projective test that also indicated progress, we are further reassured. If, in addition, there are some major behavioral changes in the patient's life, such as being able to graduate from college after failing out of many other colleges previously, this may be further evidence that the intervention is meaningful. To repeat: no one of these indices alone would be sufficient and of course we can't always have all of the indices working uniformly in the same direction; we would therefore need to develop some fairly acceptable pattern of indices.

There are a number of other factors that we might want to consider in our evaluation schema. First, we will want changes to be relatively enduring and not due to any such effect as the Hawthorne; then, we might be particularly concerned that the changes be of a large qualitative type—for example, children progressing as much as three years in their reading scores in six months. In evaluating a service we may want to consider some of its direct effects and indirect effects, its manifest results and its latent effects. For example, the doctor treats a patient and the patient gets well, but the context of the entire relationship makes the patient feel dependent and mystified; thus, it may be necessary to assess interventions at a number of different levels and evaluate them accordingly. Every human service intervention is imbedded in a context and has many meanings beyond its direct manifest goal. The open classroom can be assessed in terms of its improvement on the learning of children, measured by a variety of indices as suggested above. But the whole context has many other latent messages. In many cases this open classroom is a preferred intervention not necessarily or only because of a presumed effect on the learning of children but because of the concomitant values it expresses. For example, it is an approach that is involving of the children, drawing on their inner abilities, encouraging independence and expression. If these values are desired, the technique may be positively valued for these reasons, rather than its supposed manifest role in improving learning.

We tend to assume that the things that work fit our positive values and that things that we like also work. Thus, we are surprised when an adolescent youngster teaching an elementary school youngster obtains considerable success by punishing the child or threatening the child with the loss of lunch period if he doesn't learn something by 12 o'clock. Frequently such approaches may be successful, but we don't like them because of their latent implications. We don't want children to learn in this way, which is perfectly all right, so long as we don't believe that they can't possibly learn by any other methods beside our own approach. What we are saying, then, is that in the evaluation of any human service technique or intervention, it is important to distinguish the direct effect on improvement in health, mental health, or whatever from the more indirect consequences of the technique, the way it is presented or imbedded, e.g., the *place* such as the "school without walls" or neighborhood service center, the associated relationship, whether it is cooperative, collegial, or whatever. By confusing these dimensions, we not only fail to measure the more indirect dimension, which may have more far-reaching, long-range effects, but we often confuse the two dimensions and automatically assume that they are working in the same direction; or—and this is the more typical pattern illustrated in the various new approaches to consumer control—because the approach fits our value framework (e.g., there is consumer involvement), we automatically assume that the effectiveness of the service is thereby improved. This, of course, may be true, but it requires more *direct* evaluation procedures, utilizing multiple indices.

Finally, in the human services there are special evaluation questions related to the fact that some approaches are good for some people (and some groups) and not for others. Individual differences, style differences, and subgroup differences are extremely important. The open classroom may work very well for some kinds of youngsters, particularly those who already have a developed interest in learning, and yet it may be very inappropriate for other groups; the contact curriculum may be a complete waste of time for youngsters who are deeply involved already. Role-playing may be a useful approach with some children and may be contraindicated with others. Some teachers may use games very effectively while others function better with a more structured lesson. This is not to say that everything works, but there are many paths to Rome, many different approaches and styles that may be effective. This adds further to the evaluation problem.

REFERENCE

Campbell, D. and Fiske, D. Convergent and discriminant validation by the multitrait–multi method matrix. *Psychological Bulletin*, 1959, **56**(2), 81–104.

CHAPTER 5

Social Values and Mental Health Practices

LERNER'S THESIS is that the mental health professional's disavowal of psychotherapy with poor and Black people represents a defensive allegiance to the faulty assumption that the poor, particularly the Black poor, are too inept verbally and lack sufficient impulse control to make effective use of psychotherapy. She avers that the continued practice of offering the poor therapies other than psychotherapy is based, really, in the conflicted value system of the practitioner. Rather than looking at these conflicted values, therapists continue to cling to the assumption that poor people cannot profit from psychotherapy, even though there are cohesive empirical data that sharply contradict this assumption.

It is argued in the paper that the practitioner's capacity to conceptualize and implement appropriate psychological treatment of those poor people needing psychological services often is clouded and tainted by prejudiced and, in some instances, racist views of poor people. It is pointed out that the usual alternative treatments suggested for the poor often emphasize behavioral control rather than the freeing of inherent potential. In this emphasis on order rather than treatment, the mental health field's approach to the poor is more 17th century- than 20th century-oriented.

It is clear in our society at large that we seek to control the aims and behaviors of Black people. It is also clear that this control orientation is a defensive action to guard us against our anxious concern that unknown dark forces will dissolve those things we value; Black people have come to symbolize those "dark forces" (Kovel, 1971).

Lerner suggests that we recognize and change the dynamically determined control orientation in our professional dealings with poor and

Black people. She clarifies the point that psychotherapy is aimed principally at providing occasions in which people might maximize their individual potentials; it is aimed at eradicating internal barriers to this potential.

Lerner cautions that when these internal barriers are contributed to by problems in the individual's milieu (including the prejudice of the therapist!), the problems in the milieu must be directly confronted. In Lerner's experience, the therapist's failure to recognize his or her own conflict in social values and racial attitudes is significantly related to the therapist's disrespect of the poor or Black client's personal autonomy and, consequently, is related to therapeutic failures.

REFERENCE

Kovel, J. *White racism: A psychohistory.* New York: Vintage Books, 1971.

Is Psychotherapy Relevant to the Needs
of the Urban Poor?

BARBARA LERNER

Is PSYCHOTHERAPY—not behavior modification, crisis counseling, reality therapy, or any of the other currently fashionable adjustment techniques, but old-fashioned, inner truth seeking, one-to-one relationship therapy— relevant to the needs of the urban poor?

Most administrative proponents of community mental health and many self-appointed advocates of the poor are convinced that the answer to this question is a resounding, unequivocal, and long overdue "No." Therapy, of the sort specified above, is, according to these "new look" mental health experts, ineffective, impractical, reactionary, and obsolete: ineffective because it doesn't work, impractical because it takes too long, reactionary because it is hopelessly middle class, and obsolete because it antedates the new technology of specialized, prestructured programs and techniques.

This paper is an attempt to challenge that view a second time. My first challenge is summarized in a book called *Therapy in the ghetto: Political impotence and personal disintegration* (Lerner, 1972), a book that reports the results of a 5-year research and treatment project, an intensive study of the effects of one-to-one relationship therapy on a group of clients dominated by so-called untreatables: severely disturbed, lower class, urban Black people.

Results indicate that such therapy was highly effective with these people, as measured by client's ratings, therapist's ratings, blind analyses of projective test data, and independent measures of behavioral change. These positive changes, sufficiently dynamic to show up on the Rorschach and valid enough to be consistent across four different points of view, were achieved in a very practical amount of time—i.e., on an average, in less than 30 hours of face-to-face contact. Individual psychotherapy for the poor, the severely disturbed, and the discriminated against is, according to these results, neither ineffective nor impractical. It works—in a reasonable amount of time and for a not too horrendous cost.

Is this hard evidence likely to make a significant dent in the prevailing negative view? I think not; not even if other researchers and therapists promptly replicate these positive findings with new samples in new settings. In this area, positive evidence alone is unlikely to prevail, because the initial reaction against psychotherapy by community mental health proponents was not based solely or even mainly on clearcut negative evidence but on a set of assumptions about the urban poor and about the larger society of which they are a part. These assumptions, in the minds of many, constitute a deeply motivated and complexly overdetermined belief system and, when facts fly in the face of such beliefs, it is the facts that are likely to be overshadowed and submerged.

That being the case, I do not plan to reiterate in this presentation the facts of my research, which are reported in detail in my book (1972) and in two subsequent articles (Lerner and Fiske, 1973; Lerner, in press). Instead of going over previously reported research, I would like to challenge the prevailing negative view of psychotherapy for the poor from a different angle, i.e., by taking a more searching look at the assumptions and beliefs that lead so many workers to conclude, with or without evidence, that psychotherapy is reactionary and obsolete and should be replaced by new approaches and techniques.

The basic argument here is that therapy is an intrinsically middle-class method, hopelessly unsuitable for poor people and, especially, for minority group poor people because it is incompatible with their needs, values, and life-styles. At first glance, this seems like a criticism of therapeutic ethnocentrism and a respectful defense of the right of poor people to follow a different but equally acceptable cultural drummer. On closer scrutiny, however, the respectful note turns out to be very faint indeed.

Consider, for instance, the features of therapy that are thought to make it intrinsically middle class. Therapy is thought to be unsuitable for the poor because it provides delayed rather than immediate gratification, because the rewards involved are abstract and intangible rather than concrete and specific, and because it relies heavily on verbal communication—talk rather than action. As such, it requires of its clients a capacity for planful impulse control, an appreciation of ideas as well as of things, the ability to collaborate actively in defining problems and working out solutions, and a reasonable degree of verbal facility—all capacities that the poor, along with children and animals, are thought to lack.

Thus, inherent in this common critique of therapy is a view of poor people that constitutes either a clear denigration of them or a rather startling rejection of the most basic and universal adult human values. For a few troubled younger professionals who seem to be rebelling against responsibility itself, the latter may indeed be the case. For the vast majority of mental health bureaucrats, however, the former is really the point. These practitioners seem to regard the poor as a "species" of remedial people; what they are defending is not their right to be different but their "right" to be inferior and to be treated as such—to be given immediate tokens rather than help in reaching long-term goals, concrete cookies not clarifying concepts, and minutely structured chores instead of broad decision-making powers.

Is there any validity to this view of poor people? I think not. I think, in fact, that it is as preposterous as it is prevalent and that the supposed evidence to support it, the endless reports purporting to document so-called "cultural deprivation," are largely a product of the failure of large numbers of middle-class professionals to really communicate with poor people or to comprehend the harsh realities of the social situation they are struggling to deal with.

Elsewhere (Lerner, 1972), using examples of actual cross-class and cross-race interaction analysis, I have written about the very real verbal skills and impulse-delaying capacities of the poor in general and the Black poor in particular, and I have attempted to show how and why middle-class observers often fail to perceive these skills and capacities. An example of impulse-delaying capacity prevalent in urban ghettos is the widespread participation in that form of gambling known as "playing the numbers."

First, and most obviously, "playing the numbers" requires that one forego the opportunity of obtaining a small, immediate, concrete reward—purchasing something to eat or drink or wear—in favor of the possibility of obtaining a large, delayed reward—one that exists, at the point of purchase, only as an abstract, conceptual, and very remote possibility. The fact that large numbers of poor people do quite consistently opt for the latter reward over the former should, in and of itself, give pause to those who so confidently assume that the poor have little capacity to delay impulse gratification. Surely, it would be fatuous to dismiss the evidence here by arguing that policy wheels are also white middle-class inventions, intrinsically incompatible with the "culture of poverty."

To the middle-class mind, however, the real question is likely to be: If the poor have this capacity, why do they tend to manifest it only in such "inappropriate" situations—i.e., in illegal gambling games, where the odds are overwhelmingly against them—and not in legitimate and "realistic" life situations—e.g., in school and on the job? To my mind, and I think to the minds of many poor people, the answer is simple. Playing the numbers requires a minimal investment and offers the hope of a maximal pay-off. True, the odds on winning are depressingly low, but, for the poor, given the profound inequities in the opportunity structure and reward distribution system of this country, the odds on "winning" in the legitimate world's games are often as low.

The real difference is that in games legitimatized by the larger society, the investment required of the poor is maximal and the pay-off, usually a nonunionized manual job at subsistence wages, is minimal. Given this situation, it is understandable that many poor people play society's games only when their own survival is at stake and turn to alternative games of their own devising whenever the brute force of survival pressure is relieved.

If the foregoing analysis is correct, what is needed to improve the situation is real and profound social change—a basic alteration in the monetary distribution system of this country to create real equity, real openness, and real opportunity for the poor. The corollary to this conclusion is that there is little need for the widespread use of techniques like behavior modification and reality therapy to train and/or pressure disadvantaged people into playing more docilely and consistently with the loaded dice society hands them. Given real opportunities in a really fair game, most poor people will use the basic psychological and social skills they already possess to develop whatever additional specialized skills are necessary to take advantage of those opportunities. This has already happened in areas where real opportunity exists—e.g., in sports and in entertainment—and the same pattern should emerge when real opportunities are created in other areas—e.g., in business and in industry. On the other hand, if there is no basic change in the status quo, no amount of skill training is likely to have much impact, no matter how sophisticated our training methods become. Opportunities create skills; skills, in and of themselves, do not seem to create opportunities.

Let me make the point and the connection here even more explicit: the poor look like "remedial people," lacking in sense, skill, and capacity only if one assumes that society is basically open and equitable and that their failure to achieve success and their proneness to mental disorder is a product of their own inadequacies and deficits. Conversely, if one assumes that our society is grossly inequitable and significantly closed for many, then the social behavior and the psychological problems of the poor make perfectly good sense without the necessity of assuming them to be different from the middle class as to be lacking in elementary adult human capacities like verbal ability and impulse control. Put another way, one might say that the poor are different from you and me because their situation is different, but they are not, after all, Martians.

Being fully human and being confronted with a formidable array of socially imposed obstacles to the expression of their full humanity, the poor are forced to either deny their humanity or to engage in an exhausting, unequal struggle against the manifold obstacles that limit and deny its expression. Because the struggle is so unequal and because most poor people are still battling alone rather than as members of organized groups, they tend to lose more often than they win. Repeated failure experiences of this sort are, initially, a result of social impotence not psychological deficit, but such experiences are conducive to a sense of psychological impotence, which is ultimately conducive to the development of an overlay of actual psychological impotence.

People who have been reduced to this state and/or people who have responded to their situation with a variant of the "you-can't-fire-me-I-quit" stance by defensively denying their humanity rarely need behavioral training in basic human skills. Neither do they need to learn to regard the recurrent crises their disadvantaged position makes them subject to through Panglossian eyes as "growth experiences." It is, in fact, no more desirable for the poor to accept the devastatingly frequent, externally imposed crises that play havoc with their lives and minds than it was for Dr. Strangelove to learn to love the bomb and stop worrying.

What poor people reduced to a state of psychological impotence usually need is a restoration of their sense of personal power, which will ultimately allow them to join with their fellows in an organized group struggle for social change—one in which they will be less vulnerable and more effective. Generic psychotherapy is fully compatible with social change because it is an attempt to restore personal power—self-understanding, self-control, self-direction, and self-esteem—through the development of an honest, empathic, egalitarian relationship with another human being, the therapist.

The poor, being fully human, are in actuality fully receptive to the development of such relationships if they are offered to them by therapists with the necessary qualities. In my own previously cited research, the therapist quality that, above all others, appeared to best differentiate between effective and ineffective therapists with disadvantaged clients was the genuineness and depth of the therapist's commitment to democratic values, his respect for his own autonomy and that of others, and his steadfast rejection of authoritarian control and direction, no matter how benevolent its guise.

Professionals with such values make good therapists and, also, good advocates of meaningful social change. The poor need both types of service and from the same sorts of people, people with a genuinely democratic and not an elitist or authoritarian set of values, people who can help the poor in their efforts to define and implement their own goals and to deal with both internal and external obstacles to their achievement. Alas, many professional advocates of genuine social change feel compelled to reject the validity of psychotherapy because they think that it is necessary to choose between the two, that a focus on internal change precludes one on external change.

In actuality, internal change is only incompatible with positive external change when the internal change agent, the therapist, disrespects his client, pressing blindly for change in the direction of adjustment to an unsatisfactory status quo rather than focusing at least as heavily on the releasing of personal creativity. Psychotherapists who help to restore personal power and to release creativity are contributing to basic change, not opposing it. Conversely, social therapists who attempt to manipulate social forces and conditions so as to compel greater conformity are hardly change agents in the positive sense, even though they focus on externals rather than internals.

Think about it, please: would Richard Cloward or George Albee really have more in common with Elton Mayo or, for that matter, Gerald Caplan, than with, for example, Frantz Fanon who was, among other things, a psychotherapist?

REFERENCES

Lerner, B. *Therapy in the ghetto: Political impotence and personal disintegration.* Baltimore: The Johns Hopkins University Press, 1972.
Lerner, B. Democratic values and therapeutic efficacy, in press.
Lerner, B. and Fiske, D. W. Client factors and the eye of the beholder. *Journal of Clinical and Consulting Psychology,* 1973.

Part III

Models for Service Delivery and Program Planning

CHAPTER 6

Mental Health and Social Systems

SCHLESINGER offers a practical model of mental health intervention that is aimed at alleviation of mental disorder via correction of deviancy-producing characteristics in large-scale social systems. The model is justified on the basis that clinical (i.e., individual-focused) methods alone have been shown only to reduce prevalence of mental disorders, leaving incidence figures unabated. Schlesinger illustrates his model with concrete steps by which the mental health professional can move from individual- to system-directed efforts.

The appeal and utility of the model for mental health practitioners may depend on whether mental health practitioners are motivated to move away from their traditional dyadic relationships with clients. Central to this question is the concept of power. As Schlesinger suggests, among traditional mental health practitioners, the valued and sought after power base has been provided by professional organizations in which guild considerations have been quite prevalent. In this arrangement, the practitioner has been accountable primarily to his own professional reference group. This kind of power orientation has been manifested over the years between psychiatry and psychology in interdisciplinary fights over professional, territorial prerogatives.

In another chapter in this book, Billingsley points to the deleterious effects of a professional power orientation on mental health practice. He suggests that mental health professionals continue to neglect the study of social organizational and social value precursors to individual mental disorder. He further suggests that this neglect is self-serving in that it protects mental health professionals from explicit and critical awareness that they covertly share the investment of other social institutions in accruing to themselves uncontested institutional power.

Schlesinger's model is antithetical to the traditional mental health disciplines' concern with power. In his focus on deviancy-producing factors in society, power is considered in terms of the power of systems and advocacy groups to change deviancy-producing institutions. Power derived from professional identity and expertise is to be shared openly in interdisciplinary and community teams that work conjointly to correct social ills underlying individual ills.

Community Mental Health from a "Change-Agent" Point of View

LAWRENCE E. SCHLESINGER

THE THEORY, resources and power of community mental health programs are obviously in a state of change. Practitioners have noted a shift from traditional mental health practice focus on individual patients to the area of social and community action (Hersch, 1972). Surveys of these efforts and their consequences are provided elsewhere in this book (Reiff, Chapter 2; Wolpe, Chapter 11).

The inability of mental health funds and professional skills to support a clinical approach to high prevalence problems has been described by Glidewell (1971, p. 144). These resource shortages have resulted in attempts to supplement traditional roles by such devices as the development of paraprofessional training and utilization of patients as treatment adjuncts (Goldberg and Kane, Chapter 8 of this book). Attempts are being made to increase the capability of parents, teachers, nurses, social workers, general practitioners, etc. to deliver mental health services (Caplan, 1973). New organizations manned by nonprofessionals have been developed in conventional mental health programs and in related drug abuse programs. Finally, the resource gap has stimulated innovative programs in which mental health projects are being reconceptualized as "planned interventions in a social system" (Glidewell, 1971; Murrell, 1973).

These changes in concepts and staffing patterns are accompanied by striking changes in the role and social organization of the mental health practitioners. Diagnostic skills for assessing the impact of social system variables on mental health vary considerably from individual diagnosis. Social system interventions also require different action skills. The social relations of the practitioner, especially his power, also change. As he moves from clinical practice to community action, his task of sizing up the problem and acting must be shared with others in the community in a process Glidewell (1971, p. 146) calls "planned collaborative social intervention."

The success of these efforts to develop, demonstrate, and diffuse an innovative social systems technology for alleviating and preventing mental health problems is by no means assured. It depends in small part on having a road map to guide the efforts (assuming that sufficient vehicles and energy are around to attempt the trip!). This conceptual map has two parts—program content and organizational requirements. First, an explicit description needs to be made of the differences between individual, group, and social system problem-solving orientations. Second, we need to describe the social organization of the community mental health program for carrying out "planned social interventions." Let us examine, first, the movement from individual to group to social system perspectives in community mental health.

MINI-, MIDI-, AND MAXI-PERSPECTIVES IN COMMUNITY MENTAL HEALTH

As practitioners, we need a way of looking at our own activities that will give us increased perspective on what we are doing. Our approaches are fairly predictable if we know the way our minds are trained to work. We tend to see the world in terms of different size units such as:

1. Individuals.
2. Groups.
3. Larger social systems.

Most of us have a mini-perspective, focusing on the individual client or his family. Some have a midi-perspective and tend to think in terms of people with common problems (e.g., the problems of Appalachian whites). A few of us have a larger societal perspective. We may have reached the point of diminishing returns in applying the mini-perspective to mental health problems. At least we need some way of examining our own perspectives to see:

1. How mental health problems can be diagnosed, and how treatment or preventive interventions developed at each level.
2. Which level perspective we are working on.
3. How the other levels influence us in our work and how we might influence them.
4. How any concrete behavior can be fully understood by a combination of all three levels.
5. How there are emergent properties at each level. A small group is more than a collection of individuals. An organization is more than a set of divisions, and a society is more than a collection of institutions. Each level has its own distinct characteristics.
6. How the academic disciplines on which we rely for basic information operate at different levels.

7. How we can increase the flexibility of our approaches by adopting a perspective more suitable to the problem, even if less suitable to our biases and training.

The following table suggests a model for understanding the problem-solving perspective we use as professionals. Of course, there are more than three perspectives as we move from individual to social system. However, three are proffered for simplicity of illustration.

Table 6-1   Mini-, midi-, and maxi-perspectives.

Problem Analysis	Mini- Clinical	Midi- Group	Maxi- Social System
Locus of problem	Client	Client group	Social deviance in client group, Institutions relations
Conception of problem	Client in trouble, Crisis	Prevention and crisis intervention	Modes of deviance: Inadequate resources, External stresses
Target of change	Client, Members of family	Client groups at times of high risk: (a) Milestone program (b) Crisis intervention program (Prevention and crisis reduction)	Social System: Client, Families, Institutions, Communities, Laws, Insurance Companies, Agencies
Intervention mode	Clinical, Individual treatment	Agency, Mass communication, Programs, Services	Client advocacy, Elite groups, Social change
Knowledge base	Psychiatry Casework Individual psychology Family therapy Rehabilitation theory	Theory of communications Attitude and behavior change Organization theory Community development	Social deviance theory Models of social change advocacy Social movement theory Planned change
Assumptions regarding change	Client and family need help to solve their problems	Programs need to be available for high risk groups	Client problems can be reduced by changing the social situation
Power base	Professional helpers	Agencies	Advocacy groups

Mini-Perspective

The individual is the locus of the problem in this perspective. The individual may be viewed as having one or more problems. Individual problems are located in the body, the mental apparatus, or action capabilities. The advantages to the practitioner and his sponsors of individual-oriented treatment programs are described by Caplan and Nelson (1973). Generally, this orientation is politically conservative.

The change target, then, is seen as the individual. The mode of intervention or change effort is aimed at changing some aspect of the person by putting the person through a program aimed at altering some characteristic. The knowledge base for the procedure will come from such sources as casework, psychiatry, individual psychology, rehabilitation theory, or family therapy. The basic assumption regarding change is that the individual needs help in solving his problems. He needs additional skills, resources, or knowledge.

The power base for the mini-perspective comes from professional helpers and organizations of these professionals. We are all familiar with the territorial ambitions of specialist groups as they move toward professionalization, demarcation of domains over which they have dominion, assertions of solidarity within the group, and competition between them and other groups over control of the territory.

Many of us have spent our lives within the mini-framework. Naturally, we have not limited our attention to individual clients or their families. We have seen the effects of the environment on the lives of our clients and have made environmental interventions as well as individual ones— getting jobs for people, providing educational opportunities, finding new places to live, etc.—but the focus of our systematic efforts has been on change in individual clients.

There are several limitations to the mini-approach. We usually assume that any reasoned and carefully observed attempt to relieve pain and distress is a worthwhile endeavor. We even feel that any systematic attempt to improve people is also worthwhile. However, a cost-benefit analysis may indicate that resources might be more effectively applied at another level. For example, the resources used to alleviate the human distress of mental retardation might be more effective if applied at the level of prevention. The resources applied to driver education might be more effective if applied to vehicle or road safety design. In general, resources might be devoted more often to changing the social and physical environment to accommodate to the individual and less often to changing the individual to accommodate to the social system.

Second, the mini-perspective becomes inadequate as the number of people requiring treatment increases and overloads the facilities and manpower. The application of rehabilitation efforts to welfare recipients may fit this overload definition. The individual approach is not an adequate response to epidemics or a socialization device for large numbers of the population, such as those involved in drug addiction, delinquency, or crime. Looking ahead in our argument, it is clear that the problem is to reduce the number of new cases that appear—in other words, prevention—by alteration of physical, biological, and social systems. As specialists in the mini-perspective, we should be very slow to offer our services to solve problems of epidemic proportions.

Finally, we need to examine the amount of change we can realistically make in the lives of our clients with the resources available. All of the evidence on change from rehabilitation, psychotherapy, mass communications, propaganda, persuasion and attitude change, political campaigns, and so forth suggest that, at best, change efforts aimed at individuals have a nudging effect. They push people in the direction they are predisposed to go. When a large magnitude of change is required for large numbers of people, we should be wary of the mini-perspective.

Summing up, the mini-perspective of individual change is limited by considerations of resource allocation, cost benefits of alternative change models, the number of persons to be processed, the degree of change required, and the acceptability of the changes by the social environment. Despite these limitations, many of us continue with the same old finger-in-the-dike attitude in the face of floods. (Some psychiatrists and psychologists, we are told, have solved the flood control problem by shifting their energies to a more limited target—wealthy neurotics.) The mini-perspective—intimate, personal, and based on effective human relationships—is an important rehabilitation activity, but cannot bear the complete burden of community mental health.

Midi-Perspective

If the clinical perspective is inadequate for some problems, what can be done? The midi-perspective moves from individual clients to client groups (in the sense of people with similar problems) as the locus of the problem. Client groups are characterized in terms of the similarity of their problems, their readiness for change, and their capability of change. Client groups may be children with developmental problems, first offenders, parents of newly diagnosed epileptic children, the newly widowed, handicapped adults first entering the work force, etc. In general, the client groups consist of clearly identified populations who have reached a milestone in their lives, a point usually thought to constitute a crisis.

The problem is conceived to be one of prevention of anticipated difficulties or reduction of the stresses caused by a crisis. Changes in our lives, changes in jobs, occupations, residence, etc. are sources of stress. We have learned that the more serious these changes, the more physical and emotional illnesses people suffer. As a consequence, people need to learn to cope with anticipated changes—the institutionalized person returning to the community—or to reduce the impact of the environmental crisis—the birth of a severely retarded child.

The targets for change are client groups at times of high risk—a milestone program based on anticipated crises in people's lives or a crisis intervention program based on the predictable stresses. To deal effectively with larger numbers of people at lower costs, the intervention mode shifts to programs and communications designed and tested to meet specific purposes. Innovations in this area abound—hot-lines for the younger population, suicide prevention centers, methadone treatment, training in behavior modification for parents of autistic children, information and education programs dealing with a variety of problems. New resources are provided and existing resources are rearranged to meet the needs of client groups.

The knowledge base for these programs shifts from an individual orientation to theories of communication, attitude and behavior change, and socialization. The assumption regarding change is that programs need to be available to high risk groups. The power base shifts from professionals to agencies and organizations.

With the advent of new problems, such as drugs, or increased recognition of old problems, such as suicide, we see the emergence of new client groups, a new set of services, and a new set of people advocating the cause of their groups, seeking resources from the environment, and developing innovative change programs. By taking on new clients in innovative ways, these agencies and their personnel rise to power in the mental health movement without going through the older channels. In addition, we recognize the difficulty of established agencies to develop and implement innovative programs. The new programs usually arise from outside of the existing mental health establishment.

Maxi-Perspective

The social system perspective sees as its problem the production of deviants or deviant behavior by the system. The more narrowly the system defines the bodily, mentally, and behaviorally "normal," the more deviates there will be. The conception of the problem in this perspective is not the person who doesn't fit, but the deviant-producing system. Questions are raised such as: Are there too many sources of stress? Is inadequacy of resources a common problem? The forms of deviance can be bodily, mental, or behavioral. If children fail in developmental tasks, the problem is viewed as one of socialization, adequacy of resources made available at early ages, and design of social and learning environments.

The target of change, in other words, is the fit between people and the social system. Just as human factor specialists try to design equipment to meet the requirements of the human operator, social system designers look at the adequacy of our social designs.

The intervention mode is to search for change leverage in the social and physical environments that will increase the degree of fit between the environment and the legitimate needs of people. It attempts to increase the options available to people for learning, developing resources, and living effectively. The rate of innovation in this area is comparatively slow. In the mini-perspective, as we learned through psychoanalysis, there are some techniques of unlocking the past of an individual and freeing him up to more creative anxiety-free behavior. We have not yet learned to unlock our historical past, to reshape our organizations and institutions to meet the needs of their inhabitants. The knowledge base in this area is developing deviance theory, theories of social change, social movements, planned change—these are examples that come to mind. In general, the assumption regarding change is that client problems can be reduced by changing the social situation.

The power base in social change shifts from professionals and agencies to advocacy groups. Our problem becomes three-fold as we move from the mini- to the maxi-perspective. How do we learn to identify the mental health problems in our current social arrangements, to recommit ourselves to new goals, and to develop the leverage for social change?

ORGANIZING FOR COMMUNITY MENTAL HEALTH

The section above outlines the changes in problem-solving orientation as we move from the individual as the target and medium of change to pathology as the target and the social system as the medium of change. These changes in conceptual orientation both change the content of mental health projects and have striking consequences for the kinds of people needed, their knowledge, resources, and skills. They have even more startling consequences for the kinds of linkages the staff of such a mental health program will have to one another, to their clientele, and to the community in which they work (Lippitt, Watson, and Westley, 1958).

Signs of such changes are emerging in current mental health services and in alternative and innovative delivery systems. To so illustrate, let us sketch the human organization of a community mental health program that attempts to (1) serve the needs of individuals with severe and critical problems, (2) develop programs aimed at high risk groups, and (3) identify and intervene in dimensions of community life that may critically influence mental health. These latter interventions may be concerned with altering some specific aspects of community life or participating in the psychosocial design of new communities (Murrell, 1973).

Membership Issues

The knowledge, resources, and skills of psychologists practicing in mental health are predominantly in the clinical or mini-perspective (Cowen, 1973; Glidewell, 1971). Many have been learning new skills as they are confronted with new tasks that require understanding of community dynamics and social forces.

As mental health teams move toward social system efforts, we can expect considerable change in the kinds of people who participate as well as their motivations and capabilities. It has been surmised that the typical psychologist is more influenced by the good will and approval of his peers than by the target population affected by his work (Caplan and Nelson, 1973). However, as the client and community increase their decision-making roles, the mental health practitioner becomes more dependent on consumer good will and approval. When an organization becomes more community-centered and results-oriented, we would expect practitioners to move increasingly from intra- and interpersonal concepts and skills to skills in group dynamics, social systems analysis, conflict management, group leadership and member skills, community organization, principles of planned social change, etc. (see Bennis, Benne, and Chin, 1962).

The decision to join and work with a mental health project will be influenced by such anticipated rewards as:

1. Joining an exciting and worthwhile program.
2. Increasing involvement and influence in the community.

3. Learning new skills in community dynamics and planned change.
4. Exploring and extending our skills and abilities.
5. Working with outside consultants and participating in training activities to enhance community and planned change skills.
6. Working with community members and agencies in a peer-colleague coworker relationship.
7. Learning in intimate detail how the community operates.
8. Learning to confront and work with conflicting interests.

This view of the motives and skills of the mental health practitioner is obviously different from that of the current specialist role in a bureaucratic organization. However, this kind of motivational orientation has a number of difficulties associated with being in an innovative role in a nonbureaucratic organization. Members of the mental health project may be frustrated by their inability to produce rapid and significant changes in the community, the apparent apathy and lack of cooperation of clientele and community, or hostility and competition from other interest groups. They may have unreal expectations about their own leadership ability, the visibility and status of their efforts in the community, opportunities for personal influence and power, and so on. The many difficulties that beset innovative programs in human services have been described in detail by Sarason (1972).

Team Development

Mental health personnel concerned with social systems change will tend to work in project teams (Schindler-Rainman and Lippitt, 1972). When tasks are routine and can be divided into subtasks, the organization is typically bureaucratic with people assigned to parts of the task. Non-routine tasks typically require project teams (Bennis, 1966). The skills that the team needs will depend on the nature of the change project, community dynamics, the history of related efforts, the linkage of the change project to the host agency, and the need for adequate team leadership. These teams of professionals from different specialties, nonprofessionals, and community members will need to learn to mesh their knowledge, ideas, resources, and abilities, to develop achievable goals, and to work together to reach these goals (Collins and Goetzkow, 1964). The ability to work effectively on team projects will thus be a significant skill component as mental health develops a social technology for reducing mental health problems by social interventions.

Working with the Community

Community involvement will obviously be necessary in a program that aims at reducing the casualties inflicted by the social and man-made environment. As Hersch points out (1972, p. 750) pathogenic conditions within the community are beyond the management of the individual patient-practitioner relationship and require manpower skills and resources greater than that customarily associated with mental health professionals. As the mental health program moves from the confines of the cubicle to confront the social, political, and economic forces of the community, practitioners will need conceptual clarity in guiding these relations and providing an understandable and effective role to play in the community.

There are at least three ways that the mental health team can work with the community in a social system change project:

1. *Diagnostician and Problem-Solver.* First, the team can view the community or some aspect of it as a "target" to be changed. The project team collects information, develops a sense of need for change, and formulates change objectives and strategies for moving the community in desired directions. This style establishes the team in the role of expert and, perhaps, manipulator. The team can perform in this way alone, or with allies in the community who are sympathetic to the objectives.

2. *Data Collection—Feedback to Community.* Another pattern is for project teams to collect information and organize it for feedback to the community. The data are a kind of mirror enabling the community to examine its own state. The process of study and feedback, sometimes called "action-research," enables participants to get a sense of themselves and their community, of their shared goals, dissatisfactions, and ideas about what needs to be done—setting a process of change in motion (Sanford, 1970).

3. *Process Helping.* The project team can help relevant persons and agencies in the community perform all of the processes described above from data collection to institutionalization of the change processes. Since community members are rarely experts in social systems analysis and change, they can be helped considerably by people who are more skilled in the process of planned change. The project team will need to decide how it wants to operate, to examine its potential for helping the community, to assess the community potential for change, to establish effective working relations with the community, to develop plans and resources for change, and to implement the plans.

Develop Effective Community Relations

Mental health-community relations have been polarized around the issue of community control or "ownership" of the mental health activity by the community. Obviously, programs need to be more responsible to local needs and to the local cultural context. However, opening the board of the program to local "leadership" runs a number of risks, enumerated by Hersch (1972). Local "leaders" may not be representative of the community, may tend to represent their own self-interest over community needs, and may be hostile to the staff.

These issues of community relationships cannot be avoided, but they can be dealt with more effectively if the staff has a strategy for building community relationships. This strategy may be defined briefly as contract negotiation; it involves a process of developing mutual expectations that include the joint exploration by staff and community of such issues as:

Who are the staff members?   What is their professional training, resources, and skills? What is their level of commitment of time and energy? Both parties need to look at the degree to which the staff would be expected to respond to immediate requests for service and crisis interventions as opposed to having a longer-range goal. All those involved should be clear about staff motivations. Is the staff level and source of commitment congruent with the community needs?

Are staff skills, style, and orientation appropriate? Is the staff committed to working for change at the individual, group, organizational, or community level? Is the staff committed to any substantive issues? Both parties should establish that their interests, needs, and desires in this respect are congruent.

Can the staff be trusted by the community? Unless the members of the community trust the staff, their capacity for making useful interventions is severely limited. These questions need to be examined directly and openly in establishing a contract.

Who is the client?   The program will need at least two kinds of help from the community people whose approval is needed, and the program will need people to help with the work. First, they will need the support, approval, and legitimization of the project by community leaders. They will need assistance in the diagnosis of community pathology and the implementation of social actions designed to reduce the conditions.

Community clients may be individuals, groups, agencies, or subgroups of people in the community. Particular attention needs to be paid to the selection of client groups, for these alliances will determine how the mental health program is viewed by the rest of the community. If its alliances are all with "establishment" agencies, it will be viewed as conservative. If it allies with more extremist groups in the community, it will then be perceived as extremist. It is unlikely that the program can serve the needs of all of the political and social forces in the community or find "representative" allies. It should at least be consciously deliberate and selective and recognize the consequences of alternative choices.

Whenever possible, contractual relations should be developed with all of the individuals in staff and client groups. However, this is not always feasible and the contract will have to be worked out by legitimized representatives.

The role of the staff will be an emergent one and cannot always be spelled out to the client groups in great detail initially. There are predictable factors that can be outlined from the beginning: the amount of time to be spent, expenditures of money, degree of responsibility and accountability, and the nature of the working relationship need to be discussed and agreed upon. The client group also should be clear as to the work or tasks to which they are committed and any provision for assessment or evaluation of progress.

In general, all of the collaborating individuals or organizations who are working with the mental health project should participate in spelling out their rules, expectations, and the relationships between the different parties. This emphasis on the deliberate negotiation of a contract between the staff and community and the insistence on being explicit about issues of motivation, skills, substantive commitments, trust, tasks, and so on, will not eliminate the problems. However, this "process" orientation is analogous to the kind of contract developed by practitioner and patient as the basis for their working relationships; it is just as basic to effective community interventions as to the dyadic helping relationship.

In summary, this chapter has sketched the shifts in problem-solving orientation and social organization of a community mental health project as it moves in the direction of social systems analysis and collaborative planned interventions. The sketch may provide some direction for workers moving into this new territory.

REFERENCES

Bennis, W. G. *Changing organizations.* New York: McGraw-Hill, 1966.
Bennis, W. G., Benne, K. D., and Chin, R. (Eds.). *The planning of change.* New York: Holt, Rinehart and Winston, 1962.

Caplan, G. *Support systems and community mental health.* New York: Behavioral Publications, 1973.

Caplan, N. and Nelson, S. On being useful: The nature and consequences of psychological research on social problems. *American Psychologist,* 1973, **28**(3), 199–211.

Collins, B. E. and Goetzkow, H. *A social psychology of group processes for decision-making.* New York: John Wiley, 1964.

Cowen, E. L. Social and community interventions. *Annual Review of Psychology.* Palo Alto, Calif.: Annual Reviews, Inc., 1973.

Glidewell, J. Priorities for psychologists in community mental health. In C. Rosenblum (Ed.). *Issues in community psychology and preventive mental health.* New York: Behavioral Publications, 1971.

Hersch, C. Social history, mental health and community control. *American Psychologist,* 1972, **27**(8), 749–754.

Lippitt, R., Watson, J., and Westley, B. *The dynamics of planned change.* New York: Harcourt Brace, 1958.

Murrell, S. A. *Community psychology and social systems.* New York: Behavioral Publications, 1973.

Sanford, N. Whatever happened to action research? Paper presented at the American Psychological Association, September 1970.

Sarason, S. *The creation of settings and the future societies.* San Francisco: Jossey-Bass, 1972.

Schindler-Rainman, E. and Lippitt, R. *Team training for community change: Concepts, goals, strategies and skills.* Riverside: University of California Press, 1972.

CHAPTER 7

Federalism and Funding of Mental Health Programs

SINCE THE LATE 1940s, mental health professional training and research have been funded heavily by federal government agencies. Since 1965, this funding has been extended to Comprehensive Community Mental Health centers. These centers were designed to increase availability of services to all segments of society, particularly the poor. It is too early to make definitive judgments about the viability of such centers to help meet the mental health needs of poor people. Even so, there are signs that the federal government and, in particular, the current Administration is radically changing the conceptual and fiscal relationship of the federal government to mental health programs. It appears that this change will sharply decrease available funds and programs for the mental health care of poor people.

Foley's paper clarifies current Administration fiscal policies in terms of their bearing on planning for and funding of mental health care. His paper highlights the apparent advantages and pitfalls in the Administration's attempt to shift programmatic and budgetary control from federal to state and local agencies. In particular, Foley suggests that the current Administration is moved, on philosophical grounds, to shift responsibility and accountability away from federal agencies and toward local constituencies. Foley makes the point that this philosophical commitment (the New Federalism) is joined by Administrative and Congressional concern that too much money has been spent too unreflectively on poorly defined mental health programs. The proposed solutions are to sharply curtail new federally controlled expenditures (e.g., to stop building and staffing community mental health centers), to trim certain existing federal aid programs (e.g., Medicare and Medicaid), to advise the states on how to obtain revenue-sharing funds to retain the best of what has been demonstrated in federally controlled programs, to deemphasize hospital care in favor of ambulatory services, and to encourage the use of insurance to cover mental health illness.

Some of the possible dangers of the proposed changes are reviewed by Foley. Specifically, in the proposed rearrangements, the definitions of mental illness and mental health services are being shaped by political forces, which are primarily concerned with cost accounting. Also, the emphasis on insurance coverage may force an arbitrary and artifactual distinction between mental health problems and social problems, with coverage being allowed only for the former. Furthermore, the workability of the proposed shifts depends on political bodies having the good will and ability to develop effective mental health programs. To pinpoint the possible danger of uninformed local agencies determining mental health programs, Foley gives us an example of a state-run mental health plan that is consistent with the New Federalism and that failed due to lack of expertise in planning.

It is clear that politicizing the process by which funds are made available (e.g., having to bid and compete for revenue shares) and separating out social problems as uninsurable will mean dramatically fewer services being available to the poor. Thus, though Foley gives suggestions about how to get the most out of the New Federalism, in order to protect the interest of poor people, programs of political advocacy that are not wed to the New Federalism are needed urgently. Suggestions for such advocacy are given in this volume by Schlesinger.

National Trends in the Financing of
Mental Health Programs

HENRY A. FOLEY

SINCE 1784, there has been a continuing debate about the proper federal and state role in the delivery of mental health services. The nation has moved from total neglect of the mentally ill to Dorothea Dix's state mental hospitals, which later became asylums, to the federally funded community mental health centers of the 1960s. The present trend is to cease support of direct service and training, but to continue funding research, innovative programs, and technical assistance. State governments continue to support mental health care within and outside hospital institutions. While private insurance enables more people to receive care, local communities are demanding more public resources requiring more money. This climate provides the opportunity for those with a stake in America's mental health to negotiate priorities for support from public and private bodies. Negotiations should be based on relevant data concerning the need and demand for mental health services and data on effectiveness of current service delivery systems. We also need to understand the conceptual and fiscal relationship of the federal government to mental health research, service, and training programs. Under the Kennedy and Johnson Administrations, priorities in mental health programs were categorically set in Washington, with the states in an ancillary role in regard to services. The national mental health lobbies set the mental health agenda. Particularly influential on the federal level were the National Association for Mental Health and the Committee Against Mental Illness, along with their allies on the important Congressional committees.

Conversely, the current federal influence (the New Federalism) in mental health under the Nixon Administration is to delegate authority and leadership to the states with the federal government in an auxiliary role providing guidance and categorical funding or uncommitted funds by means of revenue sharing. The New Federalism is a type of economic federalism, which has been defined (Wallace, 1972, p. 17) as:

> A public sector with both centralized and decentralized levels of decision-making in which choices made at each level concerning the provision of public services are determined by the demands for these services of the residents of (and perhaps others who carry on activities in) the respective jurisdiction.

In the New Federalism the aim is for less federal control, more state and local discretion to plan programs, and funding these programs via revenue sharing. This Administration has stressed that state and local government officials are better able to solve the people's problems on the basis of the priorities that exist in their communities, and that a program of revenue sharing will provide state and local authorities with the power to use federal tax funds in locally devised ways.

The current Administration's position is that if a state or local program is a good program, the states or municipalities should be able to find available resources for that program. Based on this position, the President and Executive Branch recently have recommended to Congress that no new federally funded community mental health centers be started, and current commitments be honored only until fiscal 1980. This recommendation highlights the intent of the New Federalism, which is to minimize the role of direct federal support to programs and to mandate primary authority for health care to the state level.

In the case of the community mental health centers the Administration has stated that their success has been sufficient to justify state assumption of their costs. If states are reluctant to allocate their limited resources to CMH centers, it is because of a failure to demonstrate sufficient value to the legislators.

Revenue-sharing funds have been provided by the state and local Assistance Act passed by Congress in 1972, called General Revenue Sharing. The act provides $30.1 billion to states and localities for the years 1972–1976. One-third of the funds are destined for the use of state governments; two-thirds of the funds will be for the use of local jurisdictions. While revenue sharing would appear to be a logical source of financing for mental health care, it has remained relatively unutilized for support of mental health programs.

Revenue sharing will not be a panacea for the problems of funding mental health programs. Many other social service programs, previously supported by the federal government, are also requiring the insufficient revenue-sharing monies. Alternative sources of funds, such as Medicare and Medicaid, are being defined to limit their support of community-based mental health services. Congress, for example, despite its political differences with the Administration, has cut significant funds from the allocations for mental health programs authorized before 1972. An analysis of the recent budget history of the Department of Health, Education and Welfare is instructive. During the past six years, the total fiscal growth of HEW has gone from 21% of the federal fiscal budget to 35%. HEW's fiscal outlay in 1966 was $21 billion. Today it has grown to $93.8 billion. This growth reflects the inclusion of programs authorized in the years of the "Great Society," especially the Medicare, Medicaid, and social service programs (Titles IVA and XVI of the Social Security Act). In addition, the inflationary rate in the medical and social services sectors continues to have a significant impact on government expenditures.

This Administration and the Democratic Congress have demonstrated concern about the spiraling economic demand that has resulted from the uncontrolled growth in the health fields. Specifically, the concern is about Titles IVA, XVI, XVIII, and XIX of the Social Security Act. Since both Titles IVA and XVI involve uncontrollable costs to the federal government, Congress placed a $2.5 billion ceiling on these social service programs in 1972. Unless additional revenues are forthcoming to permit further growth, Titles XVIII and XIX—the health programs—will be severely limited. The first phase of restrictions on the Medicare and Medicaid programs are contained in Public Law 92-603, passed in the last session of the Congress.

With the new programmatic and financial emphasis on state responsibility, and with restrictions on Medicare and Medicaid, the federally supported expansion of direct and indirect mental health services to the poor is being curtailed. One alternative to direct federal or state support of mental health lies in private, group, and government insurance programs. What is currently available as health care under these programs will serve as a backdrop against which to analyze the consequences of the New Federalism approach to the mental health care system.

INSURANCE COVERAGE

In essence, the current insurance strategy, discussed inside and outside of government, emphasizes both private insurance for the middle and upper classes in our population, and a public insurance approach for persons in the lower income brackets.

Historically, mental health care has been provided chiefly through public monies. However, in the last two decades mental health coverage increasingly has been provided in health insurance plans, both private and federal. There are two types of private insurance policies—group and individual. An estimated 82.7 million persons are covered under group policies and 43.5 million under individual policies. Mental health coverage is more limited under individual than under group plans.

With regard to individual health insurance policies, the great majority of policies exclude all coverage for mental illness or provide benefits for a much shorter period than for general illness. The few policies that cover mental illness provide benefits in both general or mental hospitals.

The individual policy costs depend upon the amount that the insuree is willing to pay and on his previous medical history; no coverage is provided for preexisting conditions. Premium rates for group policies are determined by the size of the group insured and its experience ratings; preexisting conditions are not excluded from coverage. Similarly, in Medicare and Medicaid coinsurance, deductibles and copayments are set by the Congress and the individual states; preexisting conditions are not excluded from coverage in these public programs.

Generally, it may be said that the coverage for the mentally ill who are privately insured is certainly uneven and often inadequate. For some of those who are without any private health insurance, there are the public programs supported by the federal and state governments, specifically Medicare and Medicaid. The benefits of these programs are carefully defined, and a working knowledge should help in understanding the government's involvement in insurance support of mental health and its consequences for program support.

MEDICARE (TITLE XVIII)

This act provides benefits toward the cost of (1) inpatient care in a participating psychiatric or general hospital, (2) further care in an extended care facility following hospitalization, (3) home health care following hospitalization, and, on a supplementary voluntary basis, medical insurance. Physicians' fees are not covered. Cost of drugs are covered while the patient is in a hospital or extended care facility. A person 65 or older who is entitled to monthly cash benefits under either Social Security or Railroad Retirement is automatically covered. Eligibility for other persons over 65 is determined by local Social Security offices.

A benefit period (formerly called "a spell of illness") begins on the first day a patient receives covered services as an inpatient in a hospital or extended care facility. It ends after he has been out of the hospital or extended care facility for 60 consecutive days. He may be discharged and readmitted several times during a benefit period.

Inpatient Hospital Services

Medicare provides a maximum 90 days per benefit period subject to initial $68 deductible and $15 per day coinsurance for the last 30 days and an additional 60 days during lifetime subject to $30 per day coinsurance. Hospitalization in a psychiatric hospital is limited to a lifetime maximum of 190 days. While there is no lifetime limit on treatment in a general hospital, if a person is a patient in a psychiatric hospital at the time coverage begins, a reduction is made in days covered in the first benefit period. If a person is in a general hospital undergoing psychiatric treatment when coverage begins, no days are deducted from the first benefit period unless, immediately prior to his entitlement and within the same spell of illness, he has been diagnosed and received treatment in a mental hospital for the same illness.

Post-hospital Extended Care

Up to 100 days during a benefit period after at least three days hospitalization are covered; the patient pays $7.50 a day after the first 20 days. There is no coverage for care in a facility that is primarily psychiatric. A certified, extended care facility provides intensive care for persons who no longer need the complete range of hospital services.

Post-hospital Home Health Services

Up to 100 home visits a year by health workers to a homebound patient for treatment of the condition for which he was hospitalized are covered, providing his doctor certifies the need and establishes a plan of treatment within 14 days of discharge. Services of a mental health center can be covered only if the center is part of a participating general hospital, medical clinic, or home health agency, or is certified as a psychiatric hospital. A participating home health agency is an agency—not primarily psychiatric—that has been certified as meeting specified Medicare standards for care; these may be visiting nurses associations, health departments, or a mental health clinic that is affiliated with a certified home health agency.

Medicare Medical Insurance

For a $5.60 monthly premium, this supplementary, voluntary plan pays 80% of reasonable (usual and customary) charges for covered services after a patient meets a $50 deductible each year. Psychiatrists' reasonable charges while a patient is hospitalized are covered with no yearly maximum payment. Coverage of psychiatrists' fees for outpatient treatment is limited to a maximum of $250 per year. The same limitation applies for all outpatient treatment for psychiatric disorders by any physician.

Psychiatric services—including day care, outpatient care, and home visits—ordered by a psychiatrist, incident to his services but carried out by other health professionals under the psychiatrist's supervision, are not subject to special limitations. Up to 100 visits a year by health workers from a participating home health agency to a homebound patient are covered, providing his doctor certifies the need and establishes a plan of treatment. Mental health centers are not certified as separate providers of service. Their services may be covered if they are under the administration of a participating general or psychiatric hospital. Also, services provided under the direction of a physician and incident to his services can be covered in a mental health center setting. Drugs are paid for only when they cannot be self-administered.

MEDICAID (TITLE XIX)

Medicaid is a state-administered program of federal assistance, which every state was expected to have adopted by January 1970. Federal funds pay from 50 to 83% of the costs. Only Alaska and Arizona have at this time failed to develop state plans. People who are eligible for welfare payments from federal or state public assistance programs for the aged, indigent, blind, disabled, or families with dependent children must be covered in the state Medicaid plan. Some others may be covered at the option of the state. If a state adopts a Medicaid program, it must offer the needy of all ages the following services:

Inpatient Care

Care may be obtained in a general hospital or mental health center that is within a general hospital setting. No federal funds are available for persons between the ages of 22 and 64 who are patients in a mental hospital, a psychiatrically skilled nursing home, or a psychiatric residential care facility. A state may offer an optional benefit of inpatient care in a mental hospital for persons over 65 and those under 22. Outpatient care from a hospital administered clinic or a mental health center is provided if the services are considered hospital outpatient services.

Physicians' Services

Reasonable fees from all physicians including psychiatrists are covered.

Services in a Skilled Nursing Home

These services are covered only if the home is not primarily a psychiatric facility. In reviewing the scope and adequacy of an insurance model for mental health care, there are four basic questions to be asked:

1. Does the individual have a private insurance policy?
2. What is the extent of coverage of that policy?
3. If the person is without private insurance or other means, is he eligible for public insurance?
4. If he is not eligible, do his state or local charitable agencies provide care?

The first two questions have been summarily explored. The second two, under the New Federalism, are answerable in terms of stricter program definition and available funding.

There has been concern within both the Congress and parts of the Executive Branch that insurance coverage be expanded so that public insurance reaches the total poor population who, by definition, are not able to afford private insurance. Despite this, the Medicare and Medicaid Programs (as delineated in Public Law 92–103) are now being reformed to cover only services that fit the traditional diagnostic categories of mental illness. As a result, reimbursable services are those that are related to medical treatment and not to social services. Titles IVA and XVI formerly provided coverage for mental illness and related social services in many community mental health programs. The Congress, particularly the House Ways and Means Committee, realized that the two programs that had been budgeted at $600 million were going to cost $2.5 billion for the fiscal year. Five billion in cost dollars were projected for the next year with the distinct possibility that $9 billion would be necessary in the following year. Simply stated, the states were attempting to fund every possible social service they could. Accordingly, the states were advised to establish specific priorities because the Congress had no intention of endorsing the states' umbrella-like funding of social services. The Congress closed the open-ended nature of both titles.

During the past year, the federal message has become clear to those at the state level: The regulations and standards of the Medicare and Medicaid Programs, as well as Titles IVA and XVI, mandate the states to spell out specific care objectives in terms of identified populations. Either manual or computerized statistical systems are required to identify the patients or clients. Certain types of descriptions of what has happened to the patients will be required. This type of accountability is demanded not only in the mental health sector but also in the physical health sector. Utilization review committees are being established on an area basis so that persons can be screened before entering into hospitals where the highest cost of care occurs. Specific criteria are being set up for each type of diagnosis and each type of review committee. Obviously, there is the danger that such criteria may become restrictive and that in the mental health fields some unproductive arbitrariness will creep into the distinction between social and medical services. Elimination of most social services from inclusion in the federal programs may limit or curtail mental health strategies aimed at primary and secondary prevention by amelioration of detrimental social conditions.

NIMH Services under the New Federalism

In response to what is now becoming the largest source of funding of mental health services, namely the insurance programs, the National Institute of Mental Health has been changing. News releases indicate that the Executive Branch of this Administration aims to abandon the role of direct delivery of services through the Community Mental Health Centers (CMHC) Act. There is still a question on how the Congress will respond to this position. Congressional agreement would herald a return to the NIMH posture prior to 1963 when the main focus of the Institute was on research and training with minimal funds for the demonstration of services. Excluding the alcohol and drug programs, most of the NIMH service program is based on the CMHC Act, which expired on June 30, 1973. Although reauthorized for one year (until June 30, 1974), if Congress does not reauthorize the program on a long-term basis, NIMH (which is now an organizational triad of research, services, and training) will drop most of its service branch.

Under present planning, monies freed by discontinuance of direct active support will be made available for "marketing and development" of services. NIMH would pass on to local communities marketable concepts developed in the CMH centers program and would show local communities how they can obtain funds, not through categorical programs but through public and private insurance. Some suburban communities may be able to support CMHC's services as long as these services are tied to hospitals accredited through the Joint Commission for the Accreditation of Hospitals. In other cases, lack of federal support will mean termination of community mental health services. In any case, NIMH is moving by

Administration policy toward technical assistance to the states and to the local communities.

NIMH Support of Training Programs

There is a marked change in the type of training NIMH will support. The Institute's efforts in manpower development over the past two decades have been concentrated in the mental health care disciplines of psychiatry, psychology, psychiatric nursing, and social work. At the time these activities originated, the amount and quality of available mental health professional manpower were inadequate to meet the needs of post-war America. It was therefore necessary to underwrite extensive developmental programs in each of these areas. At the present time, although shortages still exist, professional manpower in the field of mental health is seen to have a sufficient base with which to compete in the marketplace under the normal laws of supply and demand. For this reason, the Fiscal Year (FY) 1974 budget reflects initial steps toward the phasing out of general support of institutions and individuals for training in the core mental health disciplines.

In recent years some of the Institute's training resources have already been gradually shifted into areas that lack the capacity to meet a rising demand created by the rapid growth of mental health services. Such modest efforts (e.g., New Careers) are viewed by many as successful. Because of their success and the potential usefulness of similar programs in other related areas, the FY 1974 budget includes a proposed major shift away from general support of manpower production in the core mental health disciplines. It also includes a move toward the use of time-limited projects to improve the capacity of states, localities, institutions, and service agencies to develop mental health manpower to meet local service demands, whether in professional, paraprofessional, or allied fields. This shift will involve the phasing out of most existing categorical support programs while new projects are put into operation.

In relatively short periods of time the NIMH training budget has been reduced from a level of approximately $160 million to $71 million. Under the rubric of the New Federalism, the Administration expects revenue sharing and the play of the marketplace to prevent any problems that the federal reduction might occasion.

NIMH Sponsored Research

The third major component of NIMH is research. Research support patterns remain virtually intact, with additional emphasis being placed on evaluating the effectiveness of mental health services. Alcoholism and drug addiction programs will have separate research budgets.

IMPLICATIONS OF NEW FEDERALISM FOR MENTAL HEALTH SERVICE PROGRAMS

At this time there are two major constraints in relationship to mental health care services: incomplete insurance coverage and the politics of revenue sharing. Both of these may significantly limit services for the poor and near poor.

With the provision of insurance coverage for the poor, community mental health centers could charge for their medical services and people could use their insurance to pay the charges. However, due to the limitations in current plans of insurance, either federal or state grants would be necessary to maintain support for community treatment facilities for the long-term mentally ill and for mental health education and consultation. Additionally, as ambulatory mental health care is reimbursed through insurance, there is the danger that mental health care will become the exclusive province of the medical rather than of the medical *and* social service disciplines. The danger is especially acute for the poor, where there is an interplay among personal health and social problems. By historical precedent, American health insurance has not financed social services.

Revenue sharing offers but a slim possibility that the social services aspect of mental health care will be funded. Given the predictable competition within the states for general revenue sharing, mental health care is in a precarious position. Even if mental health obtains "a piece of the revenue-sharing action" on the state level, the nonmedical aspects of mental health care are likely to be short-changed. State mental hospitals are likely to be the first fiscal priority because the hospitals consume so much of the states' budgets. The second priority of state legislators may be alcoholism and drug programs. General ambulatory mental health services that include nonmedical mental health care services may be the last mental health programs to receive state attention.

The general revenue-sharing funds are closely tied to the political processes of the states and communities; mental health people will have to become knowledgeable about their state and local political processes. That mental health services have failed to obtain significant support through revenue sharing indicates that mental health workers have yet to make a successful case in an extremely competitive fiscal arena (National Council of Community Mental Health Centers, 1973).

The local mental health constituencies must educate their state officials, legislators on the budget committees, and locally elected officials on the implications of changing federal support structures for mental health and on humanitarian options for mental health care in light of federal cutbacks. Liaison to state and local officials in authorizing, appropriating, and budgeting positions is critical if mental health services are to be satisfactorily funded.

A selling point for support of community services lies in the economic advantage of ambulatory care systems. Strong pressures for a Community Mental Health Centers Act in 1963 came from governors of the various states. They did so because their institutional systems were too expensive and were forcing increased taxation. In fact, thirteen states had passed Community Mental Health Centers Acts before the federal act. The governors came to Washington in order to obtain matching funds for the construction of facilities that the states could not afford, although some states were paying for the professional staff. In 1965 they obtained funds for professional staff from the staffing provisions of the Community Mental Health Centers Act.

Today, ambulatory care remains more economical. Presumably, the quality of such care is directly tied to availability of funds for adequate programming. Recent developments in California may provide an example of cost accounting gone astray. Twenty-four million dollars were saved by eliminating most of the state mental hospitals and by returning the patients to the various counties. One such county is Santa Clara, which now has 2000 former patients within a 10-square-block area inside the city of San Jose. One psychiatric social worker has responsibility for those 2000 patients. In Santa Clara County, as well as other California counties, there simply are not enough community mental health supports to help these former patients of state hospitals or to respond to new patients in the community. The abandonment of state mental hospitals without community care systems in place indicates a return to the period prior to Dorothea Dix's campaign for humane care of the mentally ill. Some "dumped" patients end up in the criminal justice system. Costs go up in the criminal system, but little or no care is provided.

Some watchers are concerned about this regressive pattern and have been watching the results in California with alarm. For instance, in the state of Massachusetts, the governor, legislators, mental health activists, and concerned citizens are working diligently to provide community care in the state's regionalization of mental health services. The challenges for states like Massachusetts are: (1) to set cost limits for needed services; (2) to utilize the existing insurance programs; (3) to obtain accreditation from the Joint Commission for the Accreditation of Hospitals for CMHC programs that are currently in existence; (4) to negotiate with Medicaid so that all CMH centers are reimbursed for services provided in the Medicaid program (e.g., early and diagnostic screening of children); and (5) to obtain and use revenue-sharing funds.

Since insurance reimbursement is likely to become increasingly important in support of local outpatient treatment facilities, insurance carriers will need to be persuaded that coverage of this type of case is economical. Private insurers have been losing money on their health insurance packages due to high hospital costs, and have been obtaining profits through their life disability insurance policies often sold together with their health insurance policies. *The Social Security Bulletin* of March 1973 gives a very detailed explanation of the current cost of insurance, both in the public and private sectors. The *Bulletin* specifically enumerates the health insurance administrative costs to the federal government, states, and private insurance companies. Consumer knowledge and demand prevent insurance companies from cutting back on the hospitalization benefits. Failing to clearly explain the benefit package to the enrolled population has been a traditional strategy of both the private and public insurers. For example, it is suspected that as a result of lack of information 50% of the eligible poor are not covered by Medicaid today. If all the poor were enrolled and utilized the program, Medicaid might cost as much as $25 billion or $30 billion per year, a cost not currently tolerable. Increased utilization in private insurance programs leads to higher premiums; in public programs—higher taxes. Unless it can be shown that altered benefits can include outpatient care and social service can be economical in the long run, the insurance carriers will continue to "hide" benefits and suffer utilization pressures.

Increased premiums and taxes are tolerable provided the consumer knows and wants what he is paying for. Consequently, it is important to begin to establish information and data about services in order to negotiate realistically with each fiscal intermediary and to assure the general public that the services purchased are worthwhile. The general public harbors several myths about the poor, about mental illness, and about professionals "ripping off" the federal, state, and local governments. In order to offset such propaganda and to establish responsible legitimate arguments for mental health care, justification needs to be forthcoming from the professionals, oriented to the political process. Most likely to be effective are examples of costed services, dramatic interventions, or clear indications of the value of the services to the community.

Legislators need reminding that mental health insurance coverage is absent or too limited for many of their constituents. A basic level of health insurance mandated by Congress is needed to include currently uncovered populations. Press conferences and news releases can be useful in enhancing the value and centrality of community mental health.

Finally, there is a major risk of loss of the integration of social and medical services in the mental health sector. As we move toward an insurance strategy, we move toward an exclusively medical approach in the delivery of mental health services. The insurance strategy does not allow funding of social programs. In short, fiscal resources other than insurance are necessary to support complete mental health care. In the long run, as persons become aware of the exclusion of mentally relevant social services under a medical insurance approach, they may demand a social insurance program that complements their health insurance. There are few signs, however, that such a demand will be forthcoming soon.

In the meantime, our responsibility is to insure the quality of an integrated care system and to be accountable to our fellow citizens. The political process will determine the impact of the public and private sectors, but the responsibility will remain in the hands of mental health workers to assure that the impact on behalf of our mentally disabled citizens is positive.

REFERENCES

National Council of Community Mental Health Centers Survey. Washington, D.C., February 1973.

Wallace, E. *Fiscal federalism.* New York: Harcourt, Brace, Jovanovich, 1972.

CHAPTER 8

Toward an Equitable Therapy
for the Poor

ONE OF THE prevailing explanations for the failure of the community mental health movement to make striking inroads and score major successes in the urban poor communities has been that therapists of middle-class background and value attempt to practice verbal insight therapy on patients for whom other modes of concrete and more direct action are more suited. Urban poor clients are often stereotyped as resourceless and lacking in personal value and skills for bettering their condition. The client identifies with these stereotypes, and manifests a "sick" or patient role, which, because it precludes "adequate or competent" behaviors, predetermines the failure of traditional therapy.

Challenging this premise, Goldberg and Kane suggest that successful psychotherapy requires that the recipient be able to adapt characteristics of three roles: patient, student, and healer. For the student and healer roles, the client is required to relate to the therapist and others in a symmetrical—i.e., balanced or equitable—manner. It is the authors' view that the aims of therapy (e.g., the development of interpersonal skills) can best occur in settings that permit of multiple role taking. For the urban poor with little history of equitable, successful relationships, a carefully designed program of group or family therapy in conjunction with "services in-kind" seems most likely to enhance the client's social skills, reduce emotional stress, and increase feelings of well-being. Particularly, "services in-kind to others" provide a chance for the needy client to demonstrate skills along with genuine needs without humiliation and crippling dependency.

Goldberg and Kane describe how the program for equity building and service in-kind has been implemented in their center; they mention some of the problems they have encountered, including objection to income loss by county and state agencies, discomfort felt by staff, the difficulty of finding suitable service in-kind, and the problems in providing the needed supervision for the new arrangements. Examples illustrate the principles.

It is easy to object to the authors' formulation of the urban poor client as reflecting more bias and stereotype of the liberal, middle-class mental health worker than reality. However, the end result of the initial premise seems to be a set of more equitable and balanced relationships between client and clinic, which would be seen as therapeutic under most models. This chapter provides a fine example of a community mental health clinic that has moved beyond hand-wringing or business-as-usual in an effort to make the center services useful and usable by the community.

A Missing Component in Mental Health Services to the Urban Poor: Services In-Kind to Others

CARL GOLDBERG and JOYCE D. KANE

HISTORY

Introduction

Currently, mental health programs tend to treat the social and emotional problems of the urban poor as distinct entities.* This orientation has poorly served the urban poor. Studies by Hollingshead and Redlich (1958), Minuchin *et al.* (1967), Riessman (1964), and others have convincingly documented the fact that mental health services to the urban poor are inadequate.

It is our observation that mental health services to the urban poor operate from frames of reference that are both inchoate and poorly conceptualized. It seems evident that these programs will continue to be inadequate until they are predicated upon clearly conceptualized and theoretically specifiable premises. Without systematizing a wide array of sociological, philosophical, and psychological assumptions about the urban poor into a well-defined conceptual frame of reference, mental health services are pervaded by contradictions and missing components in services.

We will attempt to demonstrate in this chapter that by designing mental health service modalities in direct relationship to a well-defined conceptual frame of reference, contradictions and missing components in services can be readily identified. Whether or not the mental health planner agrees with our conceptual scheme, he needs to realize that: "We must know what we are looking for before we find it. Theory must, therefore, precede treatment methods. Without theory, our methods can be successful only fortuitously. With partially successful methods, we get at best partially successful results" (Goldberg, 1970, p. 14).

---

*An example of this is treating the urban poor client in sessions dealing essentially with intrapsychic issues with little or no attention to the basis of current social stress. Living in a vermin-infested apartment is sufficient reason for a child's nightmares.

The mental health agency described in this paper is the Laurel Comprehensive Community Mental Health Center. The Laurel Center is the administrative and service center of the Northern Mental Health Team of Prince George's County, Maryland. The overall charge of the Center is to provide comprehensive mental health services to a highly diversified population of about a quarter of a million people. Even though this catchment region is not an urban area, it has many of the problems and characteristics of the two metropolitan centers in whose corridor it is situated. Poverty is not a major problem for most of the citizens of the area. Nevertheless, there are a number of poverty pockets in this part of the county, whose mental health needs have not been adequately met.

The Need for Innovation in Mental Health Services

The concept of community mental health that many of us espouse, but perhaps few of us practice, requires an active involvement of both community agents and recipients of services in the implementation of mental health programs. In our opinion, a sincere effort to significantly involve the urban poor in mental health services does not require large amounts of financial support. Indeed, the required expenditure may be less a matter of money than a need for the mental health professional to employ ingenuity, creativity, and a willingness to accept blurring of professional and nonprofessional roles. He also must be ready to take radical departures from capitalistic modes of thought and be willing to implement barter ("trade-off") systems of operation. In addition, he must be capable of recognizing strengths and resources in clients, so that clients may provide services to the community in exchange for mental health services made available to them.

The Laurel Center has developed a program that provides the opportunity for clients to compensate the Center and the community by contributing services in-kind for others. It is our belief that services in-kind are an important component of mental health. It is also a mental health service that has been ignored or neglected in other community mental health programs. We have found one other community mental health center that utilizes the concept of services in-kind. The Harborview Center in Seattle, Washington, had at about the same time as the Laurel Center developed an experimental program called "Payment for Services in-Kind (PSK)," which was initiated with a small number of clients. In the PSK program clients gave services to the center or the community to make up for that portion of the standard fee that they could not afford to pay directly (Sata, 1972).

In addition to the economic significance of clients contributing services to the Center and the community, a service in-kind program has, we believe, important therapeutic implications. This paper discusses the theoretical assumptions that underlie the use of a service in-kind program and the difficulties encountered in implementing the program. Strategies for further development of this program are discussed.

RATIONALE AND ASSUMPTIONS

The Role of Equity in Object Relations

Three philosophical premises order our conceptual frame of reference. First, both aberrant and emotionally disordered behavior are generated by disturbances of regulated and common systems of expected and proper (equitable) behavior between significant persons. If an individual cannot derive desired material and emotional exchanges in accordance with what he has come to expect and feel entitled to from the referent system of equity from which he operates, aberrant or emotionally disordered behavior results.

A second philosophical premise that orders our conceptual frame of reference is that reestablishment of a mutually acceptable and equitable system of conduct between persons involved in conflict and emotional upheaval tends to lessen conflict and harmonizes interpersonal exchanges. Moreover, for those individuals who have had early developmental experience pervaded by psychological exploitation and inequity in interpersonal relations, training in skillful negotiation with others is an effective ameliorative endeavor. Clearly, where the individual lacks effective negotiating skills, interpersonal accommodation—that is, the matching of his personal needs and the resources to satisfy them—becomes difficult to attain.

Third, and most important, equity can best be achieved in interpersonal relationships when the relationships are balanced. This is to say, in a relationship where one person gives more of himself than does another, the recipient becomes less valued by both the provider and the recipient himself. A balanced relationship is one in which both agents experience that they have something of value to give to the other and something of value to receive in return.

From what perspective are these premises derived? The world in which we live, devoid of the myriad of theory, explanation, and preconceived notions, is a big, booming, buzzing confusion (Goldberg, 1970). To regulate and make some semblance of meaning of this otherwise inexplicable world, all social systems (e.g., churches, schools, family units) establish normative guidelines that regulate exchanges among members. Without these guidelines, interpersonal relations would be bombarded with haphazard, chaotic, and unexpected demands and consequences.

Social systems are from time to time severely tested by inner tension and external pressures. To an ever increasing extent, churches and synagogues, the pillars of the community for generations, have sold or given up their edifices in the city and relocated in the suburbs. This situation has severely divided religious congregations. Those older members who are financially and otherwise unable to move from the city feel abandoned by their religious membership group. Still other members feel that the church or synagogue must remain in the city to remain socially relevant. The majority, who carry the heaviest financial support of the religious group, on the other hand, insist that the building and its programs be conveniently located near their suburban homes. Some social systems are better able to handle these strains than are others. Some religious congregations have been able to provide services and programs to members both in the city and in the suburbs. Others have not. Inevitably, however, breaks occur in all social systems. Deterioration of normative guidelines contributes to and further exacerbates existing conflict in the smaller units (e.g., family units) within that social system. We find in the multiple-problem families found frequently among the urban poor that standards and regulated exchanges among its members and with outsiders are not shared and do not function as they have been intended by society at large. For instance, the concept of eligibility for public welfare was intended by concerned citizens and public officials as an adequate but *temporary* provision of the necessities of life for those citizens who could not secure it on their own. Welfare, however, is rarely a temporary state of existence. There have been few serious attempts to deal with the causes of poverty in this country. As a result, it is not unusual for generation after generation of a family to be on welfare. To the taxpayer, the person on welfare is regarded as an irresponsible life-styler. Punitive attitudes and actions are taken toward the welfare family. Within this climate, members of welfare families experience difficulty communicating with one another, are unable to make meaning of their existence, and fail, subsequently, to function harmoniously.

It is our thesis that one of the most essential standards that is disturbed in these families is that of equity. The *concept* of equity (fairness) is an ubiquitous motif shaping our interpersonal styles from early in life. People tend to perceive the universe in terms of their early relationships with significant others. Their emotional being, shaped from these early experiences, is integrally related to their evaluation of the equity or inequity on the part of others in their actions toward them. Individuals who were made to feed powerless and incapable of establishing fair exchanges with significant others tend to perpetuate these feelings into contemporary relations.

Among the urban poor, these personal difficulties are exacerbated by the dearth of resources available in the home and community. The resources in short supply range from highly intelligible material commodities to more subtle psychological reinforcements and interpersonal gratifications. The individual in urban ghettos generally experiences himself as both having nothing that others value and lacking the skills to get what others have. Lacking social skills and resources, he feels incapable of freely and effectively negotiating in a fair manner with others. He feels that he can survive only by depending upon others to care for his needs, by assuming the roles of "child" or "patient." In the urban poor multiple-problem family, we find that, under conditions of social deprivation, the ever-present situational crisis is compounded by inadequate internal and psychodynamic resources such that behavioral pathology results (Goldberg, 1970).

Roles Essential to Healthy Psychological Functioning

It is our observation that persons who seek mental health services are essentially concerned with establishing equitable relationships with significant others. It is our contention that in order to develop this capacity, the client needs the opportunity to experience three essential roles in the ameliorative process (Goldberg, 1972a).

The role most ubiquitously sought by clients is that of *patient.* A "patient" is a person who, because he regards himself as "sick" or disabled, is unable to be of help to himself or others. A second role that many clients assume is that of *student.* A "student" does not regard himself as having emotional problems. He convenes with a professional worker and is quite comfortable in a psychotherapy group and other group modalities in order to learn about what happens in therapy and to accelerate what he regards as his normal psychosocial development. He is generally too intent observing interesting events in psychotherapy processes to be of much help to others. Finally, there are clients who seek the role of *healer.* The "healer" tries to demonstrate that he understands and can deal with his own problems. When in group or family therapy situations, he takes the role of "assistant therapist" and tries to compete with or win favor from the therapist by demonstrating his ability to be helpful to other group members.

It is important to realize that not only do clients assume the above described roles but that each of these three roles is essential to healthy psychological functioning at appropriate times. The "patient" role suggests that without the emotional recognition of dysfunctional aspects of our own behavior we cannot ameliorate problem areas. The conceptual scheme we have been discussing suggests that a major focus of mental health services should be to point out how the individual is seeking to achieve, maintain, or avert a position of equity with significant others in his life. This is to say, to indicate to the client how he uses the equity issue in the form of justification, rationalization, illness, and weakness to assume positions of inferiority, passivity, irresponsibility, or, on the other hand, domination, oversolicitation, and overresponsibility.

Our conceptual model suggests that the most appropriate techniques for dealing with problems of inequity are family therapy and, to a lesser extent, group therapy. These techniques are involved with the negotiation process between persons involved in significant relationships more so than in individual therapy. Individual psychotherapy in our conceptual scheme is least preferable because it involves negotiating and contracting between persons who have situationally unequal status positions. This generally serves to increase the denigrative feelings of the urban poor client, who requires something from the therapist but can give little or nothing in return. However, balance can be brought also into a one-to-one therapeutic relationship. The establishment of an equitable relationship is a more difficult task for the therapist and the patient. Individual psychotherapy is indicated primarily when a client does not have access to significant others with whom he can learn contractual skills or is so conflict-ridden that he is unwilling to accept his responsibility and right to freely contract for his ends. The role of the therapist is to aid him in moving toward taking responsibility for what happens in therapy. It begins in such small ways as sharing in the choice of appointment time.

The second role, "student," suggests that without utilizing the cognitive skills of the student we could not generalize from one life situation to the next or learn from the experience of others. If equity is an essential dimension in effective psychosocial functioning, the client must be taught directly how to negotiate for fairness in his interpersonal and societal transactions. It is not sufficient simply to seek out reasons why the client is not obtaining equitable object relations. We have found role playing and other action techniques rather useful in teaching urban poor clients how to modify dysfunctional role relationships.

Finally, the "healer" role suggests that without the experience of being of assistance to others and being recognized and appreciated for these efforts, our interpersonal relations would remain sterile and ungratifying. An expsychiatric patient has said it succinctly: "What patients want is some recognition of themselves as individuals . . . being recognized and appreciated as an individual who may have something positive to contribute" (Agel, 1971, p. 50). In the case of the Blunt family, discussed in the section on results, the mother was encouraged by the therapist to assume a "healer" role. It appeared that she had required permission from someone other than herself to take this role. In this role she served as a reinforcer of certain concepts the therapist had been trying to get the family to deal with; in addition, she gained increased status from the other family members.

Each one of us is potentially a patient; similarly, each one of us is potentially a healer. Persons who are experiencing emotional distress are not experiencing difficulty in their everyday functioning because they have assumed one of these roles but because they perseveratively maintain one role in exclusion of others. Effective mental health programs provide ameliorative experiences for their clients insofar as these programs foster a realistic integration of learning experience in which the client is enabled to let others be of help to himself ("patient"), to experience himself as being of help to others and to learn to accept others' appreciation ("healer"), and to acquire the cognitive skills needed to be an effective psychosocial agent in negotiating for himself and others' goals ("student").

Value Disparity between Providers and Recipients of Mental Health Services

The providers of mental health services to the urban poor are predominantly middle class and college educated. Their orientation toward resolution of problems is by means of rational discussion and compromise, working within and accommodating to the established social order. It is no small wonder, then, that the middle-class mental health professional's attitudes best prepare him to provide ameliorative modalities that are insight-oriented, directed toward clients who have a conscious philosophical stance toward life, are capable of abstract and symbolic reasoning, and have sufficient conflict-free areas of psychological functioning to withstand the day-to-day frustrations, tensions, and problems in order to struggle with the meaning of their existence and develop a viable sense of identity. Furthermore, middle-class oriented psychotherapy does not generally concern itself with concrete tasks and straightforward solutions to daily problems and concerns (Goldberg, 1973).

The urban poor, however, "are not readily reachable by abstract, conceptual, or symbolic intervention" (Minuchin *et al.*, 1967, p. 236). Unlike middle-class clients we attend, the urban poor "are generally action-prone, concretistic, and restricted in the use of verbal symbols. They have difficulty in producing and sustaining rational and coherent dialogue; their modalities of talking are more informative when one 'reads' behavior rather than verbal content" (Minuchin *et al.*, 1967, p. 236).

Some attention should be given to the specific communication between the middle-class professional and his urban poor client. The verbal symbols that the middle-class worker uses often do more to put the client on his guard than they do to establish meaningful communication. Too frequently the worker's symbols imply diagnosis and evaluation. It is extremely difficult, if not impossible, for a client to maintain a balanced relationship with a therapist when his behavior is regularly regarded as inappropriate. An obvious example of this is the professional's regarding the client's lack of punctuality in attending sessions as resistance and lack of motivation, when indeed time commitments have very different meanings to the middle-class worker and his urban poor client. Because the therapist "knows" what is appropriate and the client doesn't, the client's feelings of inferiority are increased.

Dumont, a community psychiatrist, finds it fascinating that studies of mental illness reveal that the incidence of psychiatric disorders is highest among the poor in all diagnostic categories except psychoneurosis—the condition most responsive to middle-class oriented psychotherapy. "Psychiatry has generated a middle-class treatment for middle-class patients" (Dumont, 1971, p. 27).

In short, the urban poor client is not oriented nor prepared to undergo the intellectual and emotional endeavors required by a middle-class worker and a middle-class oriented treatment modality. This serves to exacerbate an already inequitable and unbalanced interpersonal relationship. An effective therapist is required to give considerably of himself in helping a client come to terms with his difficulty. Ethically, the professional can receive only a fee for his services. The poor cannot afford to pay a fee. In relation to the mental health professional, he assumes an underdog, patient role, either passively or complainingly presenting his daily concerns to the professional as a perceived authority figure and waiting, in turn, to be told what to do. The practitioner, on the other hand, by training and preference, is prepared for the client to take a student role, which means in *middle-class thinking* that the client takes an intellectual interest in his problems and is willing to solve his own problems once having derived general principles in working with the practitioner.

It is no surprise then that the urban poor have been regarded by the mental health professional, in no small part in the defense of his professional integrity, as resistive and untreatable (Goldberg, 1973). These difficult clients are shuttled off to a minority group professional who is patronizingly told that he or she "understands these people better than the rest of the staff," or to a middle-class professional with a lower threshold for guilt than other staff members, or to a nonprofessional who finds himself specializing in urban poor clients.

In short, mental health services to the urban poor are oriented toward middle-class values and middle-class levels of comfort and anxiety. As a result, these clients are forced exclusively into the role of patient. Urban poor clients under traditional regimes of middle-class mental health services have little or no opportunity to experience roles of student and healer.

Community Mental Health Revolution

The community mental health movement had its impetus in humanistic and existential thought. Recognizing the importance of equity in human endeavor, it sought to avoid the serious error traditional psychotherapeutic treatment had made in creating situations of inequity, imbalance, and psychotherapeutic upmanship in work with clients, especially the urban poor. The leaders of the movement realized that the implicit status relationship between patient and psychotherapist was one that served to increase the denigration of the patient rather than role-modeling a modality in which the client can learn to negotiate freely in an effective and responsible manner.

The community mental health center rose in opposition to the traditional mental health clinic, which was a reactive clinic that waited patiently to be petitioned before dealing with individuals and families. There was little or no involvement from these clinics in treating or dealing with the environmental forces that influence the client's daily problems and contribute to the maladies of scores of other persons being seen concurrently at the clinic (Goldberg, 1972b).

Because the community mental health practitioner questioned the health of the existing normative structure in which the urban poor live, he assumed the role of a radical therapist. In this endeavor he joined with the client as a compatriot, a colleague, and a commiserator rather than as a doctor to an ailing patient. Because he recognized that immediate physical needs must take precedence over intellectual strivings, the community mental health practitioner chose to act as an advocate and teacher who brings citizens together with institutional representatives and instructs these citizens in skills in which the roles and responsibilities of citizens and their leaders may be explicitly negotiated.

The advent of community mental health, therefore, provided the urban poor with the opportunity for a second essential ameliorative experience—the role of student.

A Missing Component in Mental Health Programs: Service in-Kind to Others

The Laurel Center recognizes that the opportunity for many clients to be healers of others has been neglected in other mental health programs. The service in-kind program is designed to foster the role of healer to others for those clients who don't have the opportunity to enact it in traditional treatment modalities.

The advent of group psychotherapy and other group modalities has given many patients the opportunity to help themselves by encouraging their contributions to amelioration and the well-being of others. Many mental health practitioners are firmly convinced that the most ameliorative aspect of any therapeutic endeavor is not the insight accrued about one's own situation, or the empathy and support extended to one by others, as important as these often are. There seems to be something more basic! This is the experience of seeking to be of help to others and finding one's effort helpful and appreciated. This is therapeutic for those whom we call emotionally disturbed but who are actually emotionally impoverished. Emotional disturbance is a deprivation and impediment in growth rather than an actual entity. The so-called emotionally disturbed person has been deprived of meaningful and significant relationships with others in the home and in the community. Each of these relationships serves as a *lifeline* that sustains and maintains the individual, keeping him alive and healthy. Being of assistance to others is emotionally sustentative (Goldberg, 1972b). It restores lifelines with others. When a person performs needed social and emotional functions for others and is recognized for this, he becomes valued as a person. Concomitantly, he experiences a greater capacity for equity with others.

Moreover, unless members of the community—other clients are also community members—are involved in the care and treatment of those persons with whom the mental health clinic works and is convinced of their "cure," these clients will remain marginal and alienated figures in their own community (Goldberg, 1972b).

Unfortunately, current mental health programs do not provide all of their client populations with the opportunity to play the role of "healer." Group psychotherapy is generally a middle-class oriented endeavor. The rewards of being helpful to others are at best indirect and inferential. The urban poor client's orientation is toward concrete rewards—a direct relationship between his efforts and the reactions of the persons toward whom he is directing his efforts. He is more comfortable and skillful in performing actions than in discussing and trying to express thoughts and feelings. For example, for many of the depressed middle-aged women whom we see, life has revolved almost entirely about the home. When given the opportunity to bake a cake for a worker toward whom she feels warmly or to attend the children of other mothers who cannot afford babysitters so that they can attend sessions at the Center, her depression lifts. She experiences greater satisfaction in these endeavors than in trying, for example, to help another client understand that the anger toward her husband and children may be due to unresolved conflict with her own parents.

DESCRIPTION OF PROGRAM

The program at the Laurel Center provides the opportunity for our clients to compensate the Center and the community by contributing services in-kind for others. For example, some of our clients who have received marital counseling have compensated the community by tutoring students who are having problems in school instead of paying a fee to the Center. Housewives attend the children of other mothers who are being seen, or offer transportation to clients who have no transportation of their own.

The service in-kind program was an experimental treatment modality. Patients were not selected in a systematic way. There were several reasons for this. The program was an innovative one; we had no empirical data that would suggest which clients might best profit from the program. Our theoretical assumption, which has already been discussed, suggests that clients who experience themselves as having little or no opportunity to enact the role of "healer" in either their life in the community or in other treatment modalities would be best indicated for this program. Second, not all of the Laurel Center staff were sufficiently comfortable with the concepts of service in-kind to employ it with their clients. The selective factor, therefore, was the therapist rather than the client.

In implementing the program we felt that the client's commitment to giving services was a more important therapeutic ingredient than the economic value of the service. Therapist and client therefore discussed the client's vocational skills and experiences, his interests and avocations, as well as areas of service required in the Center or in some instances in the community. Therapist and client came to some agreement about which specific assignment would be taken and approximately how much time would be spent in giving a service. The client was then directed to a staff person, usually a secretary, to receive an orientation for the assignment. Problems the client experienced on the assignment were discussed with the therapist.

In the service in-kind program are persons who do not earn sufficient income to pay a fee and who might otherwise feel guilty and self-denigrative for getting something for nothing. There are also persons who can afford fees but whom we feel would benefit more from giving of themselves than through paying a fee. When the poor pay fees, they know that their fees are adjusted to their incomes and this reveals quite baldly their economic inferiority. If the client chooses to render service in return for services rendered him, it is likely that he can demonstrate skills and abilities of which he is proud and for which he can be admired. This serves to balance his relationship with those who are assisting him with problems of which he is less proud.

Difficulties in Implementing Program

State and County Health Systems' Objection to Program.   It was difficult selling the concept of a service in-kind program to state and county health systems that had grown accustomed to collecting fees. There are two basic reasons for these systems to resist this concept: (1) A service in-kind program results in loss of money to the state. All fees collected by the Center are sent to the state treasury, and are therefore unavailable to the Center or the community. (2) The state and county health systems view its clients as totally lacking in resources. The systems view these clients as there to be served by the health systems but expect nothing in return from them. The staff of the Laurel Center strongly disagreed with this view. We dealt with the systems' objections by simply initiating the program, writing it up on our program plans and progress reports as a therapeutic program, and giving considerable effort to specifying its ongoing effectiveness for our clients.

Staff Discomfort with Program. All of the staff seemed to agree with the concept of service in-kind. Some of the staff, however, were more comfortable with the implementation of the program than were others. This was evidenced by several staff members frequently involving their clients in service in-kind while other staff members continued to employ the traditional sliding pay-scale arrangement with their clients. The Laurel Center administration left it at each worker's option whether or not the workers would involve their clients in the program. This, in our opinion, was a mistake. If a program is efficacious, it needs to be implemented uniformly, taking into consideration foremost the needs of the clients.

Systematizing the Exchange. In a new mental health center with much to learn, finding appropriate assignments for every client was nearly impossible. Although therapists were offering the service in-kind program to patients, little creative thought had been given to exploring specifically those services that could be used by the agency and community. Consequently, more clients than could be adequately handled were sent to the secretaries for the few assignments that they could give. This proved frustrating to the secretaries, as they had too few jobs for the numbers of people being sent; in addition, it was felt that many of these tasks fell in the realm of "busywork" and did not take advantage of the creative abilities of the patients. This situation soon proved frustrating to patients and therapists as well.

Supervision of Services. It was not always clear who would supervise and work with the client on their service assignment; frequently, nonprofessional staff (e.g., secretaries) assumed this responsibility. Often they felt uncomfortable in this role. Some of the clients were difficult to work with. The nonprofessional staff felt that the therapists in these instances should have been working more closely with their clients on their assignments. The therapists, in turn, maintained that attending to their clients' service assignment would take valuable time from their therapeutic work with other clients.

RESULTS

There are countless opportunities in our day-to-day therapeutic encounters to bring the concept of balance and equity into the relationship between client and therapist. We will cite examples ranging from the brief, spontaneous response that brought about balance in the relationship, to a planned therapeutic endeavor. We will also cite some examples of actual services in-kind. We would like to state, before presenting the examples that are, we believe, successes, that there were failures. However, these failures seemed to relate to our inability to do adequate planning and followthrough rather than a lack of validity in the concept of balance and equity. Systematic study of the service in-kind program based on the concepts of balance and equity has not been undertaken; however, we do believe that such a study would yield valuable data.

Brief Spontaneous Response that Brought Balance to Relationship Between Therapist and Parent of Child Patient

Mr. Thomas was a parent without a partner rearing three children, two boys and a girl. The girl, 11 years of age, had been referred to us because of her acting-out behavior at school and some concern that she might be experiencing rejection from her father. Mr. Thomas was a late middle-aged laborer who was at this time unemployed and thus available to transport his child and to involve himself in her therapy. Once during a therapeutic hour the subject of fresh fish came up. The social worker shared that she did not know where in the area to go to purchase fresh fish. She shared further that she had a child who "loved" fish and was restricted because of diet to eating only freshly caught fish. Mr. Thomas seized upon the opportunity to offer to the worker something of obvious value to her. Mr. Thomas' subsequent letting down of his guard and openness in revealing himself following this incident produced material that showed areas where the worker was able to proceed in attempting to strengthen his relationship with his daughter.

Example of Use of Concepts of Equity and Balance in a Planned Therapeutic Endeavor

Mr. and Mrs. Blunt were clients of lower socioeconomic status who were seen at the Laurel Center upon court referral. They had three latency age children of their own. They accepted into their nuclear family three nieces of Mrs. Blunt upon discovering that the children's mother had exposed them to socially unacceptable behavior and considerable emotional and physical deprivation and now planned to give them to "friends." The Blunts scarcely had enough money to meet their nuclear family's needs; however, taking care of one's own blood relatives was a part of the family's system of values.

The Blunts, in spite of their own problems complicated by poor economic status and historical social rejection, were able to use their own natural gifts, one of which was a tremendous ability to nurture others on Mrs. Blunt's part, to provide Mrs. Blunt's nieces with excellent resocialization. This together with support from the school community enabled these children to make unbelievable progress. The problems these children brought with them began to disappear. There was no more feces smearing by the children, their enuresis ceased, and they began to practice some of the social graces (table manners, courtesy, etc.) that were part of the Blunt family's system. They also made some adjustment to the school environment. Then one of the children went to school appearing to be physically abused. Unfortunately, court procedures were initiated by the school. The court allowed the children to remain in the home and awarded the Blunts custody; however, it was stipulated that they were to be involved in family therapy. The court decision was confusing to the parents, they shared later, because it carried a conflicting message. To be brought into court in the first place was experienced by them as grossly lacking in equity. As they presented themselves to the Center for court-ordered family therapy, they expressed frustration, resentment, and acting-out behavior.

Mrs. Blunt contended that the court had no jurisdiction over her own family and refused family therapy, but did agree that two of her nieces did need help. Recognizing Mrs. Blunt's right to have some say in what happened to her family, the worker began play therapy with the two nieces. While these children had improved in many ways under Mrs. Blunt's care, there was a most definite need to work with them in establishing ego boundaries. Mrs. Blunt later shared that she felt the other niece and her own three children could also benefit from the therapeutic goals. So all of the children became part of the group.

Though the relationship between Mrs. Blunt and the agency appeared improved, she continued to behave to a great degree as though the agency's expectations and values were the only ones of importance. For example, she telephoned once to *ask* if she could cancel the therapeutic session as one of the children was sick and she had no one to babysit while she brought the others to the Center. She was helped to claim her authority in this situation. Later Mrs. Blunt shared that though she saw some improvement in the children's behavior at home, it did not equal their improvement at the Center. The worker responded by offering to hold the therapy sessions in the home. It was worked out that the sessions in the home would begin following Christmas when the children would receive new toys. It was initially agreed to have six sessions. However, the Blunts (Mr. Blunt having also become actively involved in the home sessions) wished the sessions extended to assure that they had firm grasp on helping the children to respect boundaries. Later the worker learned that there was also some fear regarding how the school and court would respond to their ending. They later were able to claim their gains, and ended.

Several months passed and Mrs. Blunt telephoned the agency, leaving an urgent message to have her call returned. The worker returned her call the next day upon her return to the office. Mrs. Blunt at first seemed aloof in her response; however, upon learning that the worker had been out until shortly before returning her call and was not showing lack of interest in the urgency of her call, she went ahead to share her reason for initiating the contact. She wished to bring one of the children into the agency again, and an appointment was set up. During the appointment, Mrs. Blunt stated that the child had shared some experiences from her early life with her natural mother. She wished to know the significance of this material and how she should handle such likely sharing in the future. She was helped with the fears she shared concerning this incident. Then, Mrs. Blunt and the worker saw the child briefly together, with the worker attempting to create an atmosphere of, "It's safe to share with us," and "We will help you deal with what it is you are sharing if we can." The child was then returned to the waiting area and Mrs. Blunt discussed what her own response in the home had been. Her response revealed warmth and sensitivity; she was helped to affirm this and asked if she felt another appointment was needed. She did not believe it was necessary to make another appointment, but said she would call the agency if she needed help in the future.

In this situation the therapist, as you have experienced in reading, actively attempted to reestablish a sense of equity and balance in this client's relationship with the agency. It was a planned therapeutic endeavor, as it was believed that the Blunts' creativity in relation to their family could not be realized until they realized again a sense of balance in their relationship with the agency. Frustrations experienced in their encounter with the agency were likely to have a negative effect on their relationship with the children, who had brought them in touch with the agency in the first place. Therefore, we struggled diligently to bring balance into the relationship with the Blunts. Comments made by Mrs. Blunt before ending tended to suggest that having experienced a balanced relationship with us helped her to assert herself in establishing a more balanced relationship with other social agencies.

Example of Service in-Kind

Mrs. Whitmore was a client who presented herself to the agency in frustration because of what she believed to be our lack of concern about what she was experiencing in a difficult marital situation. Her husband was being seen at the Laurel Center on a regular basis because of a chronic emotional problem. She and her husband were brought together for marital therapy. The husband was unable to tolerate the degree of intimacy in their relationship that Mrs. Whitmore craved. He preferred to have the relationship remain stagnant. When the wife continued to experience a thrust toward growth, he showed signs of being extremely threatened and withdrew from therapy. Mrs. Whitmore had earlier begun to play guitar for church services. She continued to do this and also began to prepare for her high school equivalency. Mr. Whitmore's behavior became increasingly more physically violent toward his wife. Thus, she was forced to move out of the home prematurely, though she had hoped to wait until completing her high school equivalency and finding a job. Nevertheless, she did find a job, secured an apartment, and renewed a relationship with her father, which had been broken while she was in her teens following his desertion of the family. She declared her readiness to end the therapeutic relationship, and we agreed that she was ready. She expressed a desire to repay the agency for its contribution to her and was told of the service in-kind program. She expressed a desire to use this service as finances were more of a problem for her now than ever in the past. She had shown in therapy that she was an extremely sensitive person and her mothering relationships reflected this. She was offered an opportunity to serve as cotherapist in a play therapy group. She was enthused and visibly moved by the confidence she realized we had in her ability to give of herself to others. Mrs. Whitmore was offered some minimal training and urged to use herself in whatever creative way seemed right to her. Without a doubt she made a meaningful contribution in numerous ways to the children who received help through the group. The most memorable contribution was through her use of her guitar and singing. She took special interest in one "hyperactive" child who showed an interest in learning to play the guitar and singing with her. Mrs. Whitmore's special interest in this youngster did wonders for his self-esteem. Moreover, Mrs. Whitmore learned a lesson about terminating relationships when the child ended with the group. This involvement in the play therapy group seemed to add also to *her* self-esteem. Mrs. Whitmore realized along with us that our agency could not have begun to help this group of children as early as it did had it not been for her assistance.

Though the value of this experience, ours to her, hers to us, is immeasurable, we are confident that payment in dollars from her for our service would have had far less value than the service she rendered in return.

Other Examples of Services in-Kind

Clients who have received marital counseling then have compensated the community by tutoring students who were having problems in school instead of paying a fee to the Center.

Housewives have attended the children of other mothers who are being seen, or have contributed to transportation for clients who have no transportation of their own.

The largest number of service in-kind contributions has been in the area of secretarial services. The value of these services in a Center with many community programs operating on a case formula budget is not hard to imagine. Thus, those performing such services soon realize their importance in the workings of the agency.

RECOMMENDATIONS

To make the service in-kind concept work in a creative and rewarding manner, it is necessary to have one person who will define areas where contributions can be made by patients and to match patients with areas of service. A coordinator of volunteers was hired by the Laurel Center to serve in this capacity, as well as to coordinate other volunteer programs. The selective factor for the program must be the client rather than the therapist. Each client must have the opportunity to participate in the program if he so chooses. To insure that service assignments have therapeutic implications, professional staff must be available to orient and supervise their clients on their assignments.

Educating the Community about the Program

A service in-kind program is a rather innovative way of viewing community resources. The public generally views lay volunteers to a mental health program as people of generous spirit who are without serious emotional difficulties. The general public needs to be educated about the concept that each of us, professional mental health worker and citizen alike, is potentially both a patient and a healer. We attempted to inform the community about our programs by writing weekly mental health columns in the local newspaper, appearing on several radio shows, conducting open houses to the community, as well as staff becoming visible and involved with several civic organizations in the community. These occasions permitted us the opportunity to discuss our programs rather informally with interested citizens.

Other Exchange of Service Programs at the Laurel Center

The Laurel Center is mandated to serve a rather large catchment area with a limited budget. Departure from capitalistic modes of operation is required to secure more mental health resources than our budget allows us. In making such departures, we utilized other modes that employed the principles of balance and equity. For example, we trained students from all the mental health disciplines except psychiatry, including mental health associate candidates, at the Laurel Center; the students in return worked directly with our clients. We supervised students in groups so that they could profit from both peer supervision and professional supervision. More students could be placed at the Center in this way than would be possible if individual supervision were utilized exclusively. We obtained the services of a group dynamics trainer from a local university who served as a process consultant to our weekly staff development group. In exchange, the senior author gave several seminars and talks at the University and provided training to students of that university. Finally, a senior staff worker at the Center trained a small group of select volunteers from the community to work with multiple-problem families. These volunteers reported that, as a result of their work with these troubled families, there were positive changes in their own families.

SUMMARY

In working with multiple-problem families and the urban poor, we must avoid falling into the trap of bifurcating mental health problems as either social or emotional problems. If we are concerned with the plight of the poor, we must first discern the issues that predicate their place in the social order. Having done this, we need to ascertain the conditions that threaten as well as advance their place in society.

Our attention on equity, negotiation, and values and the function they play in the therapeutic roles of "patient," "student," and "healer" is therefore an illustration of this endeavor. On a pragmatic level it is an attempt to devise a treatment modality and a community mental health philosophy that addresses the basic concerns of the urban poor client. To be effective, this modality must focus on the skills that will enable the client to maximize his place in society. The client must be given the opportunity to create a balanced and equitable relationship with others by learning the skills necessary for negotiating for his own ends in society.

Editors' note. The names used in this chapter are fictitious.

REFERENCES

Agel, J. (Ed.) *The radical therapist.* New York: Ballantine Books, 1971.

Dumont, M. P. *The absurd healer.* New York: Viking Press, 1971.

Goldberg, C. *Encounter, group sensitivity training experience.* New York: Science House, 1970.

Goldberg, C. Group counselor or group therapist: Be prepared. *Psychotherapy and Social Science Review,* 1972, **26**(8), 24–27. (a)

Goldberg, C. A community is more than a psyche. *Canada's Mental Health,* 1972, **20**(3-4), 15–21. (b)

Goldberg, C. *The human circle, An existential approach to the new group therapies.* Chicago: Nelson-Hall, 1973.

Hollingshead, A. B. and Redlich, F. C. *Social class and mental illness.* New York: John Wiley, 1958.

Minuchin, S., Montalvo, B., Guerney, B., Rosman, B., and Schumer, F. *Families of the slums.* New York: Basic Books, 1967.

Riessman, F., Cohen, J., and Pearl, A. *Mental health of the poor.* New York: The Free Press, 1964.

Sata, L. S. A mental health center's partnership with the community. *Hospital and Community Psychiatry,* 1972, **23**, 242–245.

Sata, L. S. letter by C. B. in Jerome Agel (Ed.), *The Radical Therapist.* New York: Ballantine Books, 1971.

Part IV

Training and Service Programs

CHAPTER 9

Community-Based Training

TRAINING PROGRAMS in the major mental health professions are characterized by a lock-step curriculum containing a mixture of academic and
practical experience. In most cases, students are led by their instructors
through a series of graded hurdles designed to prepare them for their
ultimate professional roles. In this way, novitiates are provided the same
set of values and skills as their mentors, precluding the development of
alternative perspectives or techniques. Ranz and Dunn describe a training
program for psychiatric residents that represents a radical departure from
tradition and that seems to produce the learning of new and varied perspectives on mental health and illness in a "ghetto" setting. In an interesting comparison, Ranz and Dunn analyze traditional training metaphori-
cally and compare it with their own program. Instead of hospital-based
training with a set curriculum and vertical administrative responsibility,
the alternative presented provides continuous training in the crisis center,
involvement with the client from crisis through long-term treatment, hospitalization, and aftercare. Supervision is participatory (i.e., supervisors
directly observe client-resident interactions), and the center is organized
horizontally in an egalitarian fashion.

The professional staff is expected to relate to the consumer or client on
a level and basis approaching symmetry (also see Goldberg and Kane,
Chapter 8). There is no mysticism, no truth, no right and wrong. The
resident must confront his client directly and face the problems of reality
and pathology without recourse to an antiseptic office or a shield of
professional status while promoting an egalitarian, open approach to
training. Ranz and Dunn do recognize the need for psychiatric trainees to

make sound judgments about the limits of their skill and to develop a high level of professional responsibility.

Trainers in medical schools and other mental health professions could profitably study the example presented in this chapter. The eventual value of the program has yet to be demonstrated (i.e., do residents trained in the manner described go into service careers with disadvantaged groups? What level of competence do they show? How does it compare on a cost basis with competing models?). The training represented does reflect a serious effort to make new psychiatrists capable of and experienced in dealing with mental health problems. There is nothing in the content of this new training program to suggest that its effectiveness is limited to the urban poor. However, because it was developed in an urban poor context, this program may be especially sensitive to the problems of poor people.

Training Residents in "Outer Space"

JULES M. RANZ and PETER B. DUNN

TREMONT AND Washington Avenues meet at a busy corner in the south-central Bronx. On Tremont, the neighborhood's main commercial street, the stores are crowded and there are no "vacancy" signs. Their nature and appearance clearly defines this as a transitional, poor to middle class, multiracial urban community: "The Ghetto." Within two blocks there are four Medicaid clinics, two daycare centers, and a soul-food restaurant. North on Washington Avenue there is a block dominated by three churches, two government-funded community self-help agencies, a gypsy cab company, and a busy moving firm. Sandwiched between is an assortment of declining tenements, food stores, a social club with a "keep out" sign, and a U.S. Government Post Office building that acknowledges the assistance of Postmaster General James Farley. For all the trash and broken bottles, for all the drabness, the street is alive with the movement of cars and children.

We ask you now to narrow your interest to the post office. It appears abandoned; two of the three large plate glass windows are boarded up. There is a small handwritten sign on the front door: "Open Mondays through Fridays, 8:30 A.M. to 8:30 P.M., Weekends and Holidays 10 A.M. to 6 P.M." There is nothing on the front of the building to indicate what sort of place this is that keeps such unorthodox hours for a post office. We enter the building. Near the door several desks are scattered about—haphazardly, it seems. A half-dozen people of assorted ages, sexes, and races are seated about, and there is a sense of more noise further within. Past the desks there is what seems at first to be a welter of random movement. The room itself is as big as the building: 150 feet long, 40 feet wide, and 20 feet high. The large space and the movement create a scene that resembles both a battlefield and a country fair. About 60 people are sitting, standing, and moving about within the space. A dozen desks are set up about the room and people in small groups are seated around them. Three widely separated typewriters are in action and everyone in the room can hear them. People are everywhere, congregated in groups of different sizes and shapes, in corners, between bulletin boards, and beside

115

the pillars that punctuate the room. Obviously this is not a post office, but it is hard to decide what it is. There is a lot of noise. Everything is shabby: the walls, the plaster, the chairs, the floors. Perhaps, to escape, you go toward an open door and down a flight of stairs.

As you walk downstairs you are again in another world, but no less strange. A large cavernous, unfinished (though carpeted) basement houses about 30 people. There is a large group in one corner, in a circle, moving about in some formation resembling a dance. A few tables are occupied by small groups of people talking, sewing, or staring into space. Several people are playing volleyball in a refreshingly traditional way, with a net and ball. There are a pingpong game and a game of checkers in progress as well. The scene down here is quieter, but, except for the games, it is unclear what everybody is up to. To finish your investigation, you check upstairs. In a large L-shaped room there are two quiet groups arranged in circles. One is huddled about a blackboard where words are written in Spanish; it looks like a Spanish class. The other group, somewhat larger, is seated in a circle watching a handsome gray-bearded man interview a couple. There is a video-tape camera recording the proceedings. This floor is much calmer than the other two. It is still hard to give coherency to the things you have seen on the three levels.

Let us listen to what is going on in the different groups. In the back of the main floor there are a dozen or so people in a circle. A young man is complaining that the "residents" are always dropping cases, leaving staff members to pick up the pieces. Another, looking accused, promptly responds. He does not have the time to follow new cases, what with seminars and consultation assignments. Several feet to the right there is a group of four. A middle-aged black woman is complaining about her teenage son who is sitting next to her, trying to look uninvolved. The other two are asking questions of both. Near this group a young woman, looking very sad, is talking to another young woman. The first is explaining that she is having trouble sleeping at night. Your attention is drawn away, however, because a very agitated young man is arguing with a well-dressed woman in the presence of two other men. The agitated man is talking about his apartment and his family; it is impossible to make sense of what he is saying, though each word is distinct. This group of four now drifts over to a corner, pulling some chairs with them, and falls into a discussion. The man's tones become softer and his hands begin to gesture energetically.

What do you make of all this? It is easy to place this as some sort of mental health facility, one where working in groups is the prevailing mode. The Spanish class and the demonstration interview indicate that training is integral. But there is nothing that reminds one of a psychiatric ward in a hospital or of a traditional psychiatric clinic. Furthermore, everything is remarkably public. Everyone can see what is going on; everyone can see what everyone else is doing.

This is the Tremont Crisis Center. Despite its name, it is not simply a mental health center specializing in crisis intervention. It is the locus of operation of the psychiatric residency program known as the Bronx State Hospital Track of the Albert Einstein College of Medicine, Department of Psychiatry. Though it is billed as a "general psychiatry" program, to an extent probably unequaled in the United States it stresses social and community psychiatry.

THE MEDIUM IS THE MESSAGE

In the last ten years there has been a growing interest in social and community psychiatry, and in the small group therapies that characterize its practice. Until recently it has been taught within postresidency fellowships. More and more social and community psychiatry is being integrated into the three-year curriculum of psychoanalytically oriented departments of psychiatry. The innate conflictualness of this attempt (Rosenbaum and Zwerling, 1964) and the particular attendant problems (Pattison, 1972) have received wide attention. The results of this integration have been to modify the traditional curriculum in many institutions. However the structure of training has remained essentially unchanged. It is our thesis that the practice of social and community psychiatry provides an opportunity for a different way of teaching. We are calling attention in this paper to the PROCESS of residency training. We will discuss how the process in traditional programs is generally adaptive to its stated goals. We will then present the program at Tremont, discussing how its unorthodox training structure is peculiarly adaptive to a different set of goals.

By traditional programs, we refer to those representing the mainstream of American psychiatric training. Such programs have as their goal (stated or unstated) the training of residents who will engage primarily in private individually oriented psychotherapy. The assumption underlying training is that psychoanalytic theory is the most valid and comprehensive theory of human behavior. Most supervisors are analysts or analytically trained, and analytic theory is considered the core of the residents' curriculum. We highlight four typical aspects of these programs for discussion and subsequent comparison with our alternate training model.

Hospital-Based Program

Residents rotate among the various psychiatric services of a general hospital: emergency room, outpatient department, consultation and inpatient services. The first year is generally spent seeing hospitalized patients, conceded to be the most "difficult" patients. Both patients' and residents' activities outside the therapy hours are highly structured and closely supervised. The stabilizing environment keeps anxiety within manageable limits and frees patient and therapist to pursue intrapsychic phenomena during therapy sessions. Second, it presents the trainee with a group of patients living in a uniform environment, where differences among individuals can be more "purely" studied. In the hospital setting, inner space (intrapsychic, genetic) determinants of behavior are emphasized, while outer space (environmental, here and now) determinants are equalized.

Weekly Office Supervision

Specific help and teaching about therapy occurs once a week in the supervisor's office, away from the patient and the therapy situation. This encourages reflection and understanding. This is appropriate to the theory of psychoanalysis that posits that insight is basic to therapeutic change. It also maximizes the possibility for the teacher to influence the student. The teacher's role as evaluator of the student encourages (explicitly or not) the trainee to think as the supervisor thinks.

Vertical Administration

Decisions are transmitted from hierarchical superiors to hierarchical inferiors. Alterations in the structure of the program are made at the supraresident level. This provides the faculty with the opportunity to impose checks on resident activities. It also contributes to the ethos that the resident is a junior member in a discipline that is learned slowly by listening to seniors.

Prescribed Curriculum

The body of knowledge taught is prescribed by the faculty, with alternate points of view underrepresented. This follows from the assumption that the task is to teach a specific predetermined body of knowledge. This approach is helpful to the resident alone with his patient in his office, struggling to make sense out of what is going on.

Traditional

This training format has come under attack for being inflexible and inappropriate in today's context. However, its applicability to training for traditional psychiatric practice can be illustrated with two models.

The first model is the analytic situation itself, where the patient is lacking something (understanding his own intrapsychic phenomenon) that the therapist can provide, in a process where anxiety is fostered within manageable limits (by cautious interpretation). During psychiatric training, the resident is considered to be lacking something (how to use knowledge about intrapsychic phenomena to understand patients' behavior) that the supervisor can provide, by an anxiety-provoking situation (treating psychotic patients) that is nonetheless controlled within manageable limits by the hospital structure and constant supervision. We believe the similarity is not coincidental. The experience the resident is undergoing (the training process) is as intrinsic as the content of what he is learning (analytic theory), and both are mutually reinforcing.

The second model is religious education. The aim is to have the subject internalize a set of values he must maintain in the absence of external reinforcing pressure, as for example the monk leaving the monastery. The psychiatric resident going into his private office experiences a similar lack of external reinforcers.

In 1914 Freud warned against the dangers of "wild psychoanalysis." To this day, everyone cherishes a particular story of such and such therapist's outlandish behavior. This is not surprising. The private practice of psychiatry is just that, "private." The office psychiatrist is pretty much on his own, free from external restraints in his daily work. Freud's fears have been dealt within the psychoanalytic establishment by the creation of a highly structured system of training: the psychoanalytic institute. The analyst's training is geared to provide a well-internalized theory that translates into a prescribed way of behaving vis-à-vis patients. This training model has been applied in a modified way in most psychiatric residencies. It resembles and gains support from teaching in other branches of medicine, though it differs significantly in that the psychiatry teacher rarely observes the treatment process itself. It is well suited to counterbalance the lack of structure and constraints within the therapy situation itself.

Community-Based Program

About four years ago several faculty members of the Department of Psychiatry of the Albert Einstein College of Medicine conceived of a training program dedicated to the goal of training residents who would go in increasing numbers into the public sector. This followed several years of conflict within the department, and the eventual split was seen by many at the time as an unfortunate failure of the analytic model to incorporate alternate viewpoints. The members of this group, based at Bronx State Hospital, were all conversant with the principles of natural systems theory as it applies to psychiatry. Thinking within this framework, they took aim at the typically fragmented structure of most programs (six months on emergency room duty, six months on the inpatient service, twelve months in OPD, etc.). They proposed that residents spend three years in one place, following patients from their first contact with the treatment facility, through evaluation, hospitalization if necessary, and continuing with conventional individual, family, group, or medication therapy. Traditional hospital-based programs cannot accommodate this because the patient doesn't get to the hospital ward until much has happened. Residents seeing patients in ER's can rarely follow them to the hospital because most wards are set up so as to require full-time attendance of resident doctors. Once discharged, patients rarely return to hospitals, so they must be seen, if at all, in some clinic nearer their homes. These clinics, with their waiting lists, are rarely in a position to handle immediate problems. The Bronx State proposal envisioned a community-based center equipped to handle intakes and long-term therapy, but also set up with a day hospital and, hopefully, some means to have inpatients housed part of full time in the community as well. Table 9.1 presents the assumptions underlying traditional training and training at Tremont.

The Tremont community was chosen as the site for the training program, partly because it is a section that comprises a mixed group of Blacks, Whites, Puerto Ricans, and Fordham University students—assuring a variety of teaching material, and partly because it was an area totally devoid of existing outpatient mental health facilities. It already contained a recognizable and functioning local community group concerned with matters of health, the Tremont Health Planning Council (THPC), with whom we could negotiate and thus avoid the pitfalls of "dumping" a training program on a lower class community.

It is generally acknowledged that the most effective treatment to be offered in such a community is crisis intervention. Thus, a contract was drawn up and signed by the State of New York, Department of Mental Hygiene (which provides the funds), the THPC, and the City of New York (whose Health and Hospital Corporation "owned" the turf and which provides emergency ambulance service for the area to Fordham

Table 9-1   Comparison of assumptions underlying training.

Traditional Program	Tremont Crisis
Assumptions	
Goal is to train residents who will engage primarily in private practice. ("Where")	Goal is to train residents many of whom will go into the public sector
The primary mode of therapy is individually oriented psychotherapy ("How")	The most effective modality is natural system-small group intervention
The most comprehensive theory of individual psychotherapy is psychoanalytic theory ("Why")	Natural systems theory is the most comprehensive model for therapeutic intervention
Consequences	
The format of residency training resembles the individual-oriented analytic model (Thesis of paper)	The format (process) of residency training tends to create an experience of a living, changing natural system
The contemplative stance is encouraged (Ego ideal)	The activity stance is encouraged
Natural systems is a different, probably valid but peripherally relevant theory (Attitude toward other's theoretical framework)	Analytic theory is a subsystem of natural systems theory
Success of training is measured by the extent to which resident assimilates psychoanalytic theory (Measure of success)	Success is measured by resident's involvement in his natural system—extent and quality of contribution
Intervention is most effective and relevant on individual level (Level of intervention)	The higher on the natural system continuum you intervene, the greater the likelihood of producing change (individual → family → network → society)

Hospital). The contact provided for the formulation of the Tremont Crisis Center (TCC), which would provide crisis intervention and hospitalization to the community. This center became home base for the new residency program of the Albert Einstein College of Medicine—Bronx State Hospital. The Crisis Center and residency program opened simultaneously in July 1971.

Crisis intervention is most effectively handled by a team approach, so the delivery of clinical services was organized along the lines of crisis teams, to one of which each resident was assigned throughout the three years of training. This approach dictates two important attributes of residency training as it developed at the TCC: (1) all initial patient contacts are made by the crisis team (represented by at least two members, usually one resident and one staff member), so that the resident must work very closely with staff members (who usually have less training but more experience, less money but more expertise), and (2) the supervisor participates in the crisis interviews.

Supervisor as Participant-Observer

The incoming resident is immediately placed in a situation where clinical work must be performed under the eye of the supervisor (rather than reported to him after the fact). The supervisor as participant provides an model that tends to break down traditional teacher-student boundaries and encourages the working model of "do as I do" rather than the more academic "do as I say." Working in each case with supervisors and staff members of many disciplines teaches residents to be more flexible in their approaches, as well as encourages (some might say forces) residents to learn how to work effectively with other professionals and non-professionals.

The TCC ended up in the abandoned shell of a post office largely by accident, but in many ways it was fortuitous. Lacking the traditional offices and corridors usually associated with mental health centers, staff members, residents, and faculty alike were forced to learn to deal with each other in new ways. No longer did the largest office automatically convey status—nobody had an office. Everything happened out in the open: seeing patients, meetings, supervision, training, and even courtship. This creates a distinct peculiarity, residents are encouraged to "do their own thing" but find that everything they do is being monitored by supervisors, staff members, and secretaries. No longer can the resident take his patient into his office and sometime later present an edited version of his session to his supervisor. At the TCC the supervisor is usually either right there taking part in the interview or across the room within eyesight.

The Horizontal Organization

Bronx State is a fairly typical, if somewhat flexible, vertical organization. The Hospital Director entrusts several Unit Chiefs to run each unit;

they are responsible for everything that happens in their unit and report directly to the Hospital Director. In turn, each Unit Chief appoints an administrator of each of his hospital wards, who reports directly to the Unit Chief; and so on down through the structure. Decisions are invariably made at the top and filtered down by way of memos; lower echelon people can make recommendations (or often are requested to do so) in the form of memos that pass up the ranks until a decision is made and then pass back down. This traditional "vertical" business organizational model is being challenged on a number of fronts, but nowhere does it seem more inapplicable than in community-based psychiatry. Unless the director of the program and the teaching faculty happen to believe that psychiatry already has all the answers as to how to deal with urban communities, they must provide for effective participation in decision making by all levels of the organization, including residents.

The TCC was established in the spirit of modified egalitarianism (doctors still make more money, teachers still have more status than students) and was committed to a horizontal form of organization. This is a complex, cumbersome, and often inefficient form in which small groups tend to form either permanently or temporarily around certain issues of importance to the members of that group. These groups put forth proposals that then get aired in a variety of ways—formally (in committees and in full-scale staff meetings) and informally (rumor and word-of-mouth). Reasoning, arm-twisting, sharing favors, and other forms of lobbying may be used. Decisions are made either by the entire group or by some small committee authorized by the group to review and make that particular decision.

Residents Devise Curriculum

This has several important spinoffs for residency training: (1) Lacking clear directives from on high, residents are left to make their own peace with the program and its members. The acting principle is "do your own thing," although, to be sure, this carries the additional burden that one must be fully responsible and ready to deal with whatever reactions one's "own thing" may engender in the people with whom one works. (2) Residents form their own natural grouping, and our program encourages (again, read *forces*) them to potentiate this grouping not just to T-groups, but as a pressure group of its own, which gradually becomes experienced in lobbying for its own causes. The resident becomes experienced in lobbying for his own causes. The resident becomes experienced in the ramifications of power and authority. (3) A natural outcome of all this is that residents are free (in fact, have the responsibility) to choose their own training curriculum. They plan how much and what kind of formal education they want, choose to what extent they wish to involve themselves in the many opportunities available to them through the TCC, the community, and the Albert Einstein College of Medicine (not just during their elective third year), and choose their own supervisors and teachers.

When we discussed the traditional residency model, we drew an analogy to one-to-one therapy. At Tremont, we stress family and natural system intervention and the striking thing is that life in the Center is rather similar to life in a small community (overcrowded, of course), coping with on-going change. In other words, in both residency models the resident steps out of therapy sessions into an environment that is structured to complement the goals of that therapy. In our residency, the experience of being a resident is of constant negotiation and active participation in decision making. Like a member of a small community enmeshed in his system, the resident can react to what others want of him or, as is encouraged, work for his own interests by taking stands and finding out who is allied with him. The residency itself becomes a lesson in organization and negotiation rather than contemplation.

"DOING ONE'S OWN THING" IN A "FISHBOWL"

Many people have been disturbed by what appears to be a lack of hierarchical controls on resident activities. This concern grows more out of the appearance of physical chaos than out of an examination of the residents' programs. Indeed, most residents are involved in programs that would satisfy anyone's requirements for a general residency. This chapter grew out of an attempt to understand how all the work got done, and how residents developed respectable curricula, given the lack of clear guidelines from above. This led us to consider the paradox that the resident is told: "Plan your own activities, we trust your judgment," and then must proceed to carry out most of his activities in a "fishbowl" under continual observation. It also led us to realize that the "natural constraints" inherent in the practice of small group therapy are basic to understanding the workability of the "do your own thing" ethos in our setting. Consider the following pressures intrinsic to small group therapy as it is practiced at the TCC:

Influence of the Group

First, the therapist is outnumbered, usually facing an integrated though often disharmonious group. Whatever deviant behavior brings them to the psychiatrist is usually mutually reinforced and mutually protective. The social psychiatrist often feels like a man pressing on an archway where each stone keeps the others in place. Furthermore, he often works on "foreign turf," his patient's home territory. And one additional factor is that while a patient frequently admits that he is a patient, a natural group rarely does. The end result is an overwhelming feeling of powerlessness. This is probably a realistic view of the situation.

Influence of the Cotherapist

One way to help counterbalance this sense of powerlessness in relation to the group is to bring in allies. This may be one's colleagues or a whole mental health team. "Maybe they can beat me, but not my whole gang." However, as far as a personal sense of control goes, this is a mixed blessing; while the social psychiatry trainee is now better equipped to deal with his patient, he must modify his behavior to fit in with that of his cotherapists. And, as Rosenbaum and Zwerling (1964) have written:

> Once the focus of attention has shifted from the patient as an individual to the patient as a member of a group, the psychiatrist no longer has the same feeling of professional security and superiority with his non-medical colleague as does his more traditional counterpart. Even the familiar psychiatric social worker and clinical psychologist are more group oriented than individual oriented.

Influence of the Supervisor

Once the law of privacy, integral to medical and analytical practice, is broken by bringing in a natural group (e.g., the family) and cotherapists, other options follow. The supervisor feels free to sit in or even to function as a cotherapist. Again, for the trainee's sense of control over the therapy this is a mixed blessing. He gains in his mastery and understanding of his problems with the group and his cotherapists, but he feels the presence of his advisers; his behavior must be modified to conform with their expectations. We believe that these sources of feedback during the therapy situation allow the planner of a teaching program to relax further extra-therapeutic efforts to monitor his trainee.

"ACTION" VS. "CONTEMPLATION"

It is probably obvious that our program encourages an "active" mode of practice rather than the contemplative mode of traditional psychiatry. We harness a great deal of energy that trainees in traditional residencies devote to passively and actively resisting the hierarchy. We reward and channel creativity. We allow residents to create highly personalized programs in which they are more heavily invested. In practice, we see ample evidence of this point. Administration, consultation, and community involvement are part of life at Tremont, often inseparable from clinical work. Residents play a crucial role in the ongoing development of the still highly unstructured service delivery system at Tremont. They serve on all working committees—curriculum, coordination, residency selection, personnel policy. A resident is chairman of the curriculum committee. All this activity, unfortunately, comes at the expense of the more "contemplative" modes: (1) seminar attendance, though "required," is sometimes erratic; (2) while our residents undoubtedly are more familiar with the ramifications of natural system theories, they are probably less conversant than their traditional colleagues with psychoanalytic theory; (3) while they often perform spectacular crisis work, long-term follow-up (especially in chronic cases) has less glamour and is often overlooked.

"TEACHER SHOCK"

We have also become aware of the disorganizing effect this program has had on its teaching faculty, especially at the outset. Professional teaching personnel, used to the relative solitude of hospital-based training programs, experienced varying degrees of "teacher shock," marked in its extreme cases by disorientation, powerlessness, and uselessness. The phenomenon was manifested in the entire group by a lack of cohesion (no meetings of faculty were held in the first six months, and then irregularly through the first year). Probably inevitably, when the faculty began to "get itself together" at the start of the second year, many territorial battles ensued. Nonetheless, staff and residents alike found themselves in a better position to challenge faculty initiatives because they already had active natural groupings of their own to mobilize.

SERVICE DELIVERY

What kind of service gets delivered at Tremont? Although we see our training program as radical in design, our service delivery system is remarkably traditional. The basic mode is brief, family-oriented crisis intervention and psychotherapy, featuring a walk-in service (no waiting list), frequent home visits, and efforts aimed at preventing hospitalization. When hospitalization becomes necessary or desirable, we provide this directly on our own ward with our own staff. We do not provide narcotics or alcohol detox or treatment units.

Crisis intervention, family therapy, and the newer network therapies, as well as long-term intensive individual psychotherapy, are practiced in abundance, and well, by our residents and staff. We do less well on long-term support and medication cases, although probably as well as most programs. A constant source of discouragement has been the quality of inpatient care we provide. Though probably adequate, it is far from imaginative, and often regarded as a poor relation of the more "exciting" crisis work and community consultation.

CONCLUSION: THE QUALITY OF THE TRAINING PROGRAM

What kind of residents will emerge from this program? By our own avowed goal, we should produce a higher proportion of residents going into the public sector. This will be the single most important index of success. At present, we are pleased to have 19 residents in our program in only its second year. This includes three second-year and two third-year residents who have transferred from other more traditional prestigious programs. We are continuing to attract high quality trainees for next year, both as first-year residents and as transfers into our second and third year. One resident left our program at the end of the first year. We also have been actively recruiting minority-group representatives from residency training, and have at present one Black and four Spanish-speaking trainees. All residents are actively involved in our "community" as indicated above, but on more conventional grounds they are doing well also: all see individuals, groups, families, and adolescents (most also see children) as well as participate in the on-going crisis work, community consultation, and hospitalization intrinsic to the program.

It is clear that there are many unpleasant side effects and even dangers to working in "outer space." As long as everybody (faculty, residents, staff, community) feels he has a stake in the success of our program, and a say in which direction we move, we are confident we will continue to be an exciting and effective program.

REFERENCES

Pattison, E. M. Residency training issues in community psychiatry. *American Journal of Psychiatry*, 1972, **128**, 1097–1102.

Rosenbaum, M. and Zwerling, I. Impact of social psychiatry on a psychoanalytically oriented department of psychiatry. *Archives of General Psychiatry*, 1964, **11**, 31–39.

CHAPTER 10

A Model of Service to Youth

FROM THE vantage point of ten years of scholarly and professional mental health work with delinquent adolescents, Shore offers a number of valuable perspectives. His program served disgruntled, economically deprived, socially acting-out, public school drop-outs in suburban Boston. The value of the program to those served, as compared to matched subjects in a control group, has withstood the test of a ten-year follow-up. The generality of the program to another target group (i.e., discharged mental hospital patients) also has been shown.

Even so, there is no evidence of widespread application of the program, and Shore's paper clarifies the fact that the inherent value of a service program alone does not determine its viability in the mainstream of mental health service delivery. Issues that militate against high visibility and broad use of effective programs include: (1) poor capability of formal and informal mechanisms for disseminating information about new and effective mental health programs, (2) the degree to which the program content grates against conventional professional practice, and (3) the extent to which program concepts challenge conventional social values.

In particular it is noted that practitioners have no reliable sources to which to turn to become informed about what is valuable among the rapidly increasing numbers of offerings in professional publications. Perhaps of greater significance to the low visibility of Shore's program is the fact that it requires nonconventional roles for its utilizers. For example, the "therapist" in his program frequently was required to be available at odd hours and at odd places (e.g., street corners) and to engage in unusual practices such as finding jobs and serving as a reading tutor.

Concerning values, Shore points out that the therapist accepted the client's wish and right not to be in school. No attempts were made to remotivate clients for formal schooling. Rather, their employment motivation was supported. The paper makes it clear how this orientation grates against two social issues: first, the powers that be in our society seem quite ambivalent about rendering meaningful aid to those who are underemployed and wish to improve their employability. Second, our society (including conventional mental health agencies) is oriented to youth being in school even though schools often have difficulty retaining youth with personal and/or social adjustment problems.

Shore also points out that programs targeted to the poor encounter the powerful, if sometimes subtle, conflict in our society concerning the poor. That is, as a society we seem to need to maintain some groups in poverty.

Shore suggests that correction of the forces that work against full enactment of services for the poor will require political as well as professional action on the part of the mental health specialist. A possible model for such action is provided in this volume (Schlesinger, Chapter 6).

Making Innovative Community Mental Health Programs Marketable

MILTON F. SHORE

In 1963 a colleague and I initiated a community mental health program for youth who had left high school, were chronic academic failures, and had been in continual trouble with the police (having been on probation at least once). This high risk group had not been helped by the traditional mental health services within the community and the schools. Such youth have often been called (in characteristic "blaming the victim" fashion) "unreachable," and have formed the core of major criminal activity in the community. Although the program was developed in a suburban community, most of the youth were from families in the lower socioeconomic classes. Despite its scope, the cost of the program was relatively low. The details of the program have been described in a number of publications (Massimo and Shore, 1963, 1967; Shore and Massimo, 1966, 1969, 1973). Called "comprehensive, vocationally oriented psychotherapy," its major assumption was that these antisocial "dropout" youth could be reached through a program focused around assisting the youth in finding a job in the community around which all other necessary services (such as remedial education and psychotherapy) could then be offered. The major features of the program were:

1. The services were initiated at a crisis point. Within 24 hours after the boy had left school, he was contacted and offered the opportunity to get a job. He seemed most amenable to such an offer at that time.
2. The services were not affiliated with other community agencies. The therapist was independent of the schools, clinics, or social service departments. No effort was made to encourage the youth to return to school unless he chose to do so. Instead, many alternative educational programs—such as industrial training courses, night school, and correspondence courses—were explored when needed.
3. The services were flexible. Most often the therapist and youth were not in an office but somewhere in the community doing many things together, such as visiting employers, buying a car, etc. There were

few restrictions on time and place. The therapist could be contacted at any time of the day or night.

4. Individualized services were stressed. Efforts were made to meet the individual needs of each youth. The therapist himself offered any of the services that were needed (remedial education, job counseling, or psychotherapy) without a referral being made to other agencies or departments.

5. The focus was on concrete tasks, most of which were nonverbal. An action orientation aimed at independence was emphasized with an emphasis on the development of cognitive and personal skills through activity.

The program was carefully evaluated. Not only was there an independent evaluation of overt behavior, cognitive change, and personality change over the ten-month period of intensive therapeutic work, but there have been follow-up studies two years, five years, and ten years after treatment. A group of boys in the program was compared with a group that was left to the regular community resources. Out of this study have come some 20 publications in well-known journals dealing with the theoretical, research, and practical aspects of the program. All the results show that the program was extremely effective over a long period of time.

The study has been well received by the professional community. The research element received a commendation from a division of the American Psychological Association. The work has been referred to very favorably in the literature on research in psychotherapy, treatment techniques for adolescents, new approaches for helping the poor, and many other areas. The program could even be seen as antedating by three or four years the philosophy of the New Careers Program, the National Job Corps, and the Neighborhood Youth Corps set up as major strategies in President Johnson's War on Poverty.

That does not mean that the program has been above critical comment. Many have noted that it was a small study (limited by the availability of only meager funds). Some have questioned whether the therapist (only one was used in the study) was not one of those rare charismatic persons whose qualifications could not be found in another person. Therefore, they feel the results might not be able to be replicated. Some correctly have observed the differences between suburban and urban communities and noted that the program's usefulness in urban areas has not been demonstrated.

However, despite these criticisms, all of which appear not to question the study itself but are rather directions for further exploration, the program generally has been accepted as setting a significant new direction for community mental health programs for groups of high risk. (The principles of the program recently have been found to be highly appropriate for a group of patients discharged from a state mental hospital [Fisher *et al.*, 1973]. Rehabilitation of those patients in the special aftercare program was significantly more successful than in those patients left to usual community resources.)

Yet, despite the general acceptance of the value of the program and despite its publicity, the study has had little impact on the field over the last decade. In discussing, in general, how a community mental health program can be made marketable, we can attempt to answer the question with specific reference to this particular program.

There appear to be two sets of issues in marketability—those that are related to problems in dissemination and utilization of research knowledge in general, and those related to the specific content of the program.

Studies of the dissemination of research information have found some startling results. The amount of information in the field of mental health has risen so rapidly that it has become extremely difficult to even keep up to date with material most pertinent to one's everyday activities. Therefore, those in the service area more and more have had to limit themselves to sources other than the printed page. As noted by the National Institute of Mental Health (HEW, 1971), only 9% of the innovations in mental health services have been found to be stimulated by printed research findings. Instead, the gap between practice and research (similar to the two cultures theory of C. P. Snow) has been widening as research continues to be seen as irrelevant to practice.

The publication lag also can be seen as contributing to the lack of utilization of research results. By the time results get into print (often two to three years after the project has been completed) and are available, decisions have already been made. The tempo of the field has accelerated to the point where information is almost obsolete before it is available to a large audience. Because of this, systematic efforts are currently being undertaken at the National Institute of Mental Health to promote the distribution of significant literature to practitioners as soon as possible.

But there is another general factor that prevents the adoption of innovative programs that might be of some value to service delivery—namely, the nature of the program itself. It is this content of a program that can explain why sometimes one program is adopted although it has not as yet proven its usefulness, while another program is rejected or ignored.

There were many elements to comprehensive vocationally oriented psychotherapy that appear to have prevented others from using it in whole or in part, either in an effort to replicate its results or in an attempt to broaden its applicability.

First, it was not a simple program. We did not deal with discrete variables such as those of the behaviorists. The focus, rather, was on a complex individualized approach that dealt with the concepts of needs, relationships, and flexibility, all of which are currently not in vogue in the social sciences because they are so difficult to define operationally.

Second, the services all were administered by a single person who sometimes had the role of counselor, at other times of educator, and occasionally as job locator. This way of delivering services is not the way our current service structure is conceptualized. Instead, we have been maintaining rigid boundaries between disciplines, attempting to fit those in need into our current structures rather than trying to set up any new structures that might be necessary. There is no reason why individuals who work with the "unreachable" cannot be trained in multidimensional ways so as to develop the understanding and competence necessary to respond to these diverse needs.

Third, the program challenged some basic values of our society. Some government agencies refused to share their job files because "young people should be in school." Although they were told that these youth were the ones that do not return to school, such an explanation was not adequate to gain the agency's cooperation.

Likewise, we must recognize that dealing with employment and its meaning in our current economic climate is bound to arouse considerable opposition. The response to the recent report on *Work in America* (HEW, 1973), released by the Department of Health, Education and Welfare, reveals that we do not want to take a careful, hard look at the role of employment in our society, especially the issues of guaranteed jobs, major improvements in the conditions of work, opportunities for useful work despite severe handicaps, etc.

One basic value that appears to have been challenged by this program is how willing we are to make some major changes in order to deal with the many social problems that plague us. Are we serious about doing something lasting and significant or do we still maintain a "band-aid" approach aimed at simplistic surface changes that look good but fail to deal with the major cause of the problems and to prevent their development?

What has been learned from this study with regard to marketing innovative community mental health programs?

First, the gap between knowledge production and knowledge utilization again has been found to be vast. Techniques need to be developed for more adequate utilization of relevant research findings in service delivery systems. More opportunities for personal contacts between researchers and practitioners are necessary to foster and reward innovation in the delivery of mental health services to high risk groups.

Second, there is a need to recognize that major changes in service structures are brought about through the political process. No amount of information or scientific proof in itself will bring about major changes in service delivery if they do not become part of the political machinery. An example of this is that Dr. Jerome Miller, a social worker in Massachusetts, was only able to produce massive changes in the handling of delinquent youth in the Commonwealth of Massachusetts Youth Service System when he received the strong support and cooperation of the Governor of the state. It is the professional's responsibility to recognize that he must be part of this political process, constantly making the information that he has gained available to those in political positions. It is necessary that the professional also think about the relevance of his work to current political issues, and that he join with others in political activity, using his scientific research as a resource for bringing about change. Thus, the professional's role may shift at various times from that of the scholar to that of the consultant, to that of the innovator, to that of the advocate, to that of the strategist, to that of the change agent. The marketability of his ideas, however, is dependent upon his skill in carrying out the various roles, and requires him to make available in appropriate ways material that can form the basis for important decisions in social policy.

Gans (1971) has described in detail the important roles the poor play in the total psychological, social, and economic structure of our society. He points out that some of the needs are being met in other social classes by maintaining the poor in positions of poverty. His analysis reaffirms the complexities of the problem and the depths of the resistances that can be expected when a change is brought about in services for the poor, particularly in urban areas. The mental health professional has a role in seeing that the inevitable change that occurs is built on a foundation that is humanitarian and just.

REFERENCES

Department of Health, Education and Welfare, National Institute of Mental Health. Preface to "Planning for creative change in mental health services, information sources, and how to use them," 1971.

Department of Health, Education and Welfare. *Work in America.* Cambridge, Mass.: MIT Press, 1973.

Fisher, T., Nackman, N., and Vyas, A. Aftercare in a family service agency. *Social Casework,* 1973, **54**(3), 131–142.

Gans, H. The uses of poverty: The poor pay all. *Social Policy,* 1971, **2**(2), 20–24.

Massimo, J. and Shore, M. The effectiveness of a comprehensive vocationally oriented psychotherapeutic program for adolescent delinquent boys. *American Journal of Orthopsychiatry,* 1963, **33**, 634–642.

Massimo, J. and Shore, M. Comprehensive vocationally oriented psychotherapy: A new treatment technique for lower-class adolescent delinquent boys. *Psychiatry,* 1967, **30**, 229–236.

Shore, M. and Massimo, J. Comprehensive vocationally oriented psychotherapy for adolescent delinquent boys: A follow-up study. *American Journal of Orthopsychiatry,* 1966, **36**, 609–615.

Shore, M. and Massimo, J. Five years later: A follow-up study of comprehensive vocationally oriented psychotherapy. *American Journal of Orthopsychiatry,* 1969, **39**, 769–773.

Shore, M. and Massimo, J. After ten years: A follow-up study of comprehensive vocationally oriented psychotherapy. *American Journal of Orthopsychiatry,* 1973, **43**(1), 128–132.

CHAPTER 11

Advocacy and Activism

THE TWO CASE examples strikingly portrayed in this chapter by Wolpe provide impressive anecdotal evidence that activism by mental health professionals can have an important and lasting impact on the social order. Since the consideration of psychological research data in the Brown v. Board of Education Supreme Court decision in 1954, it has become increasingly apparent that the knowledge and skills available to the mental health professional can be significant factors eventuating in social change.

The style represented by Wolpe may not be either possible or desirable for all of us. However, as illustrated in the school intervention case, the role of social intervenor requires a facile mind and good judgment. The problem situations tackled by Wolpe involved her in rapid movement from crisis to crisis. In each case quick and incisive action was demanded. Such an enterprise is not for the weak-hearted, well-meaning tinkerer. Clinical skills, especially those of observation, critical analysis of communications, recognition of feeling states, and reading of multiple level communications, seem to be essential skills for successful action. To facilitate the use of these skills, Wolpe found the process of directly confronting conflicts and the avoidance of "blame throwing" to be two major operating principles. From reading her account, it is also clear that finding and building coalitions served to constructively redirect disruptive, disorganized energy.

The second example presented by Wolpe shows that avoiding legalistic policy rules and regulations aimed at thwarting actions and efforts and facing the issues on the basis of their essential elements can help the fight against "city hall." Wolpe and her colleagues were willing to use all avenues of attack against their adversaries, including the courts, publicity, political pressure, professional associations, and direct confrontation.

Wolpe begins her presentation with the presumption that her cause is just. From there, the mobilization of her resources and those of the community follow. In these two examples, however, many other individuals become deeply involved in the on-going drama with less clear commitment or understanding of the basic moral commitment. Most readers will agree with Wolpe's personal moral judgment in the two cases cited. The problems of social advocacy become particularly acute, however, when the moral imperative is less obvious or less universally held, and when other, relatively powerless individuals are "used" for the cause. The subtlety and complexity of these problems can hardly be overstated (see Reiff, Chapter 2), but these should not be an excuse for inaction or for limiting action to complaining in respectable parlor-room conversation.

The Role of Advocacy in Community Mental Health:
Two Case Presentations

ZELDA A. WOLPE

ONE OF THE most clearly defined mental health problems in our society is White racism. It has had a lasting impact upon our educational system. Schools are embedded in invincible prejudice and dedicated to the perpetuation of the myth of the affluent White man's superiority. Such superior status can be maintained only by the continued oppression of others. Segregation of Blacks and Chicanos into ghettos is the means of stripping them of the dignity to which they are entitled, of quarantining them so that they cannot contaminate, or threaten, those in power. But the warden of a prison is imprisoned by those he must watch. Whites remain boxed in as long as they insist upon repressive measures for others. The boomerang returns to the point of origin. We must begin to focus upon justice and injustice rather than upon law and order. There can be no education, that search for enlightenment and truth, when irrational prejudice permeates our system. Our tenacious belief in our superiority is but a myth, a reaction formation to our ignorance and guilt. We must begin to deal with our hang-ups and develop ways to eliminate White racism. Mental health workers are confronted with this serious challenge that demands the pooling of our knowledge, skills, and experience in the field of human behavior if inequities in our society are to be rectified. We must dedicate ourselves to a genuine commitment to the goal of mental health for a society too long embalmed in bureaucratic resistance to human dignity and fair play. Most of us have been brainwashed into believing "You Can't Fight City Hall." The resultant hopelessness has become the rationalization for our apathy, and we are guilty by default when we accept the myth of our impotence.

Our generation of children and the minorities have the accumulated anger of past generations within their souls. They exist in a society that has always condoned greed, war, violence, and preferential treatment for a few. These nurtured seeds of violence must erupt unless we find ways to bring about change for the victimized. Riots have occurred, both in our schools and in society at large, and have been followed by governmental demands for "Law and Order." Such slogans are invented by those who are dedicated to the preservation of the status quo by further repressive measures. Armed police can stop any school rebellion, but they cannot prevent the feelings of hate that periodically must explode when injustices and inequities are continually ignored.

Two case presentations, one dealing with racial tensions in our schools and the other with the inequities behind Civil Service Examinations will be used to consider the mental health worker's role in dealing with social issues. The rationale for the manner in which these cases were handled stemmed from personal experience with individual, family, and group therapy. Much knowledge regarding human behavior has been gleaned from clinical experience and is, at least to some extent, applicable whenever human beings are in stress but resist change, even though their repetitive behavioral patterns are self-destructive and act as a deterrent to the discovery of more rewarding behavior. Whites, for example, have often failed to see how their racism has limited their own horizons and personal growth and has heightened their anxieties and fears.

Serious self-examination to resolve any personal covert racial biases is the first grave responsibility of a consultant. No White person is immunized against the indoctrination of racial prejudice that permeates American culture. The comfortable label of "liberal" is often a hindrance to deeper examination, that painful process that strips away the veneer of phony humanism and demands a total reevaluation of work-usage, ideologies, myths, past apathy, and value systems. Our current social issues are deeply rooted in our past. Only with self-examination can we become truly aware of our embedded attitudes and become free to explore new directions. It will be seen in both case presentations that the resistance to change presented the greatest challenge. The barriers to communication due to the degree of anger, frustration, cultural differences, power struggles, a polarized community, and unconscious racism compounded the difficulties and necessitated flexible strategies in order for a level of trust to develop.

A COMMUNITY IN CRISIS

In November 1970 racial incidents occurred in two junior high schools and in one high school in a northern industrial city. Six White students had been seriously injured, one having required heart surgery and the others hospitalized for possible brain concussions. The community, for the most part, was demanding police protection in the schools and had raised

$180,000 for this purpose. I, accompanied by Dr. Nathan Murillo, accepted the invitation for our consultation services and spent ten days in the community. Only the highlights of these sessions will be reviewed.

When we arrived at South Junior High School and found all doors locked, we knew the fear contained within. We walked through the tension-filled corridors to the office where the principal and some Black and White counselors were planning their strategy for the imminent explosion they had sensed. The principal let us know there would be no time for briefing, and so I asked him to bring the ten most militant White students to the office. While he fetched them, I suggested that the Black counselors leave, assuring them that following the session for Whites there would be a session for the Black militant students at which time I would appreciate their presence.

When the ten students (with an air of bullyish bravado) arrived, I initiated the session by saying, "I understand you are having some problems at this school. Would you agree?" There was a unanimous "Yes," and so I continued. "What do you think the problem is?"

The blame-throwing onto the Blacks was without exception. After their feelings were uninhibitedly expressed, we posted large sheets of paper on the wall, and a student volunteered to write down their impressions of Blacks:

1. Blacks are a different color.
2. Blacks are prejudiced.
3. Blacks are spear-shakers.
4. Blacks get mad when Whites group.
5. They think they're better than Whites.
6. They won't jump you a second time if you don't fight back.
7. Blacks stick together.
8. Blacks are two-faced.
9. They always push you around.

Out of the discussion that followed, there were two significant statements:

1. When Blacks fight they always go for your head.
2. When Blacks start to fight with a White kid and he doesn't fight back, they leave the White kid alone and they don't go after him again.

When asked if this was different behavior from Whites, one student said, "Sure! That would be the kid we'd really go after 'cause we'd be sure to get the best of him. It just proves how dumb they are!" The other students, agreeing that such behavior was proof of the Blacks' stupidity, allowed me to redirect the discussion from blame-throwing to self-examination.

I pointed out that in our experience, though Whites always insisted that every riot was initiated by Blacks, we were able to determine in many instances that Whites had provoked the incidents; we wondered whether anyone in this group was intelligent enough to see how Whites might have been responsible, at least in part, for Wednesday's cafeteria rebellion.

After much initial denial, one boy whispered, "N.K.O.," and the entire group laughed with obvious embarrassment, but none was willing to decipher the code.

I commented, "All of you appear ashamed to repeat the words, but I'm in the dark and not very good at guessing games. In practically every community we have to learn new three and four letter words. We can't communicate very well if I don't even know your words."

Finally, one student blurted out: "Nigger Killers of Oseco." I then learned that three weeks previous to our visit 30 students bused from Oseco, on all White community described as primarily racist, had marched around and around Black students shouting, "N.K.O.—Nigger Killers of Oseco." When I pursued further: "Was there a society of Nigger Killers of Oseco, perhaps an off-shoot of the Ku Klux Klan, and what did you think would be the Blacks' reaction to such taunting?" student after student stated:

"We were just kidding."

"We didn't think they'd get mad."

"Of course there really isn't an N.K.O. society!"

All of this was said with much nervous giggling and defensive jargon.

Finally, one boy said, "Well, maybe we shouldn't have done it, but that was three weeks ago. Why are they still sore?" I was able then to confront them with their unwillingness to assume the responsibility for the consequences of their behavior. I felt the anxiety lift as the focus shifted from blame-throwing to self-examination and finally to a problem-solving orientation. When I felt a readiness for them to work with the very students with whom they had been fighting, I ended the session by asking, "If the Blacks are willing to meet with you after lunch, would you be willing to meet with them?" There was total agreement that this could be helpful. They were told that they would be notified if such a meeting could be arranged, were dismissed, and the Black militant students and counselors were brought in for their session.

A close duplication of procedure revealed striking differences in the general behavior of the two groups. The Blacks demonstrated none of the giggling, were considerably less defensive, and maintained a more serious approach to their search for a solution. A list of 19 grievances was formulated:

1. Whites think Blacks are dome. (When the lists were later posted no one questioned the misspelling of dumb.)
2. Whites are prejudiced.
3. Whites blame Blacks for everything.
4. Black kids are always getting expelled.
5. Whites always win.
6. Whites think Blacks are all the same.
7. White teachers don't listen to Black kids.
8. Blacks are not believed by Whites.
9. Whites are unfair.
10. Black kids have no one on their side.
11. Whites don't want Blacks in school.
12. Whites impose their way on Blacks.
13. Whites pick on Blacks.
14. Sometimes Whites cannot be trusted.
15. Whites don't treat Blacks with respect.
16. Whites are bullies.
17. Whites kick Blacks around.
18. Whites think that all Blacks are trouble makers.
19. Whites think they're better.

Everyone became involved in the discussion of the 19 points, and when the session had to be terminated because of the lunch hour, the students suggested that they forfeit lunch since it was more important that their problems be resolved. When asked if they would be willing to meet with the Whites in a joint session after lunch, they too enthusiastically welcomed the plan.

We arranged a large circle of chairs in preparation for the session, and the students' charts were hung on the wall. When all the students had gathered along with the Black and White counselors, I asked the students to be seated. Spontaneously, all the Whites sat on one side of the circle and all the Blacks on the other. The level of anxiety was high, the Whites giggling among themselves, while the Blacks glowered at them in angry defiance—a stance they had not employed in the morning session.

Our starting point was reviewing the lists each had made regarding the characteristics of the other. I read the first statement on the White list: "Blacks are a different color." I asked: "Is there anyone who would disagree with that statement?" Both Blacks and Whites laughed, and the answer was a loud "No!"

I said, "Ye Gods! You all agree on something!" Their laughter had barely relieved their anxiety when a Black female student, considered a prime instigator of trouble at the school, said: "Wait a minute! I'm not sure I agree. The male carries the color in his genes, and since White men usually get black women, how come the babies are called Blacks?" Several Black students took up the point with such remarks as, "Yeah! How come!"

Another Black student proceeded to give a scientific discourse on chromosomes but was interrupted by a third student saying, "I don't know much about this scientific junk you're yelling about, but if that kid has any part of him Black, I'll take him. He's O.K. with me!" The group quieted down immediately, both Whites and Blacks apparently recognizing this boy's pride in being Black.

We turned to item two: "Blacks are prejudiced." I pointed out that on the Black list item two was: "Whites are prejudiced." Both Blacks and Whites vehemently protested the accusation the other had made—the Whites saying they weren't prejudiced, they just didn't like being beaten over the head, whereas the Blacks stated: "We're not prejudiced. We just hate all Whites because we have good reason!"

"Yeah! We're not prejudiced. You are!" The students batted it back and forth until a Black counselor spoke up:

"Well I'm prejudiced, I hate all Whites! I'm damn prejudiced!"

I responded to his remark by saying: "You are telling me you are prejudiced against me—you hate me—you don't trust me and, you know, I don't trust you either. We don't know each other."

He became furious, and in a loud, angry voice said, "You're putting words in my mouth! I didn't say that. I said I hated all Whites. I do trust you!"

I interrupted by saying," I'm sorry. You're quite right. I know I don't trust you. Trust, to me, can develop only after a time-tested relationship. I was assuming your definition of trust was the same as mine. I don't under-stand how you can really trust Whites when you hate them."

He said, "Well, I do trust people, and I never want to lose that."

Finally, I said, "I can only speak for me. When you said you hate all Whites, I felt you were banging a door in my face. I have a feeling if I really got to know you, I could really like you, even trust you."

He said, "I think I could like you too!"

During this heated confrontation the students remained totally silent. I asked, "Were any of you afraid we would come to blows?"

Both Blacks and Whites yelled "No!"

When I asked, "How come?" one White student said, "You're adults."

I responded, "Come now! You're selling yourself short. I think what you saw were two people who completely disagreed with each other, but we never lost respect. I knew I wanted the door left open. We might be able to learn from each other. I wasn't going to bang a door and rob myself of what could be a great experience for me if I really got to know this gentleman."

The students relaxed and we proceeded. I asked that six chairs be brought into the center of the circle and requested three Black and three White volunteers for the inner circle. The six students were to discuss feelings, attitudes, or anything else relevant to the racial tensions. If a White person in the outer circle wished to respond to a statement of a Black, he could tap out a White person and replace him in the inner circle; similarly for the Blacks. I stressed that the procedure was to lightly tap, not punch, and within minutes everyone became intensely involved. A White boy began by saying, "I like Blacks as a whole!"

This brought an immediate response from one Black young lady who snarled: "A whole what?"

Alan looked nonplussed by the question. He repeated his statement: "I like Blacks as a whole."

Dawn came down harder this time. "A whole what, damn it!" The tension was mounting.

I said, "Alan, I think you're hiding. I think you know what Dawn means."

Alan's expression became a complete blank. "No, honest! I don't know what she's sore about. I said I like Blacks as a whole."

Dawn's fist was taking shape. A Black boy came to the rescue. He looked directly at Alan and said, "Would you date a Black girl?"

Alan quietly responded, "No. Would you date a White girl?"

The Black student said, "Sure, if we hit it off."

Alan said, "Hm! Gee! Then I guess I am prejudiced!" I knew at that moment that Alan was beginning to make the grade. The Blacks had removed his mask. More important, Alan was beginning to know where he stood. He had taken a first step in honesty.

The students were tapping each other in and out so quickly that at times statements were never completed, but their total involvement could not be questioned. In his eagerness to get into the center, one Black student tapped a White who responded automatically by returning to the outer circle. This now left two Whites and four Blacks in the center. Rick put his hands to his hips and yelled, "This ain't fair. There are four of them and only two of us!"

From the sidelines, I quietly asked, "How does it feel to be in the minority?" The response was dead silence and never again a mention of unequal distribution.

The Blacks attacked the Whites with every four letter word possible. The anxiety level of the faculty had been high and rose to a peak. The teachers and counselors were certain that the group would break out into physical violence. They began to say: "Cool it"—"Watch your language"—"None of that!" I did not want the students to pick up their message and carry out a physical explosion. In order to let the faculty know that I was in control of the situation, just as a White boy was blaming the Blacks for all the problems, I said: "Wait a minute, kids! We're losing the issue. The blame-throwing is not useful. Let's do some self-examination." The students stopped in their tracks as if I had lifted a baton. The teachers relaxed and then the youngsters continued their ventilating of feelings at gut level.

A White counselor decided to get into the act and proceeded to tap out a White student. In a most contained manner that failed to mask his controlled hostility, he directed his statements to Dawn. Her tirade had been against the White students who always blamed the Blacks, knowing full well that the teachers always believed the Whites and never even listened to the Blacks. He began his speech: "First of all I will not talk to you if you are going to yell. You know it is not permitted in our school to use profanity. You will talk civilly or we cannot communicate."

My anxieties were now rising. I had been delighted with the freedom with which the children had dared to speak in the school setting. I did not want him to force them back into their boxes. Dawn was ready to take him on. She said, "Won't you admit the Black kids are blamed for everything?"

He said, "Yes."

Dawn continued: "And aren't we always being expelled from school, even if we didn't start the mess?"

Again he said, "Yes." Then he qualified his answer by adding, "Well, not always."

Dawn shouted, "You said before we're *always* blamed! How come you change it now?"

He apparently wanted to demonstrate his absolute fairness. He said, "Well, always is a little too much. It wouldn't be true, but most times."

Dawn went on: "And aren't you always taking the White kids' side? You're one of those prejudiced teachers! All of you blame us for everything that goes wrong, and you never even listen to us."

His contained anger was mounting. He used my statement, intended for the Whites, as his authority. "Didn't you hear Dr. Wolpe say that blame-throwing is unimportant? So everyone blames you, so what! You don't have to use such vile language—so they blame you!"

His controlled speech had gotten to me. I could feel Dawn's impotence to deal with this man whose seething hatred could not be hidden behind his transparent cold veneer.

I put my arm around Dawn while directly confronting him. "Did you honestly think my remarks about blame-throwing were intended for the Blacks? Are you telling this child that she has not been blamed unjustly long enough—that she shouldn't mind it—that she shouldn't even use words that approximate her deep resentment for such injustice? I heard her say you are a prejudiced treacher. You come across to me that way too."

A look of pathetic astonishment crossed his face. As if he could not believe what he heard, he puzzled, "Do I come across to you that way?"

I had a single word in response: "Yes."

His reserved attack on Dawn gave Rick the impetus to fearlessly provoke the Blacks. Once more he put his hands to his hips and snarled: "Well, I want to say something. I don't ever want to be friends with those dirty Niggers!"

I responded, "You don't ever have to be friends, Rick. You might rob yourself from knowing some pretty great people, but I wonder if you would share with us the reason that you feel this way."

Rick, in his most surly manner, said, "Yeah! I don't like getting hit over the head all the time!"

I said, "You're telling us you're scared."

Rick was furious. "I didn't say that! I ain't scared of any of them. I just don't like getting hit over the head all the time!"

I replied, "Well, I'd be scared if I'd get hit over the head." Rick broke down crying. I reached over to him and said, "Rick, you now seem more human to me. It's all right to cry."

One of the Black boys, obviously sympathizing with Rick's embarrassment over crying, said, "Lots of times when I act mad, I'm really scared," and another boy added, "Yeah! And sometimes I feel sad!"

The group was dismissed with the understanding that we would continue on Monday. As I walked through the hall, I saw two of the White boys crying and two White counselors consoling them. I was concerned that the process might be diluted. I had worked all day to get these students to remove their masks of anger and begin to deal with their fears and sadness.

Nevertheless, at the end of Friday's session I felt the students were off to a good start. We decided to spend the weekend as productively as possible in getting acquainted with the community problems. We had been surprised that none of the school officials had contacted us in order to give us some background to the current crisis that could be helpful for the planning of our strategy. Fortunately, my son, a City Commissioner at that time, was contacted by a policeman, a father of one of the White boys injured in the high school riot. He demanded that immediate action be taken for the protection of students. Realizing that he was expressing the sentiments of the White parents of the other injured boys, we requested that he have the parents and boys meet with us on Saturday at 3 P.M. We also arranged for school administrators to meet with us on Sunday at 8 P.M., specifically requesting that the Superintendent and Board Members along with counselors and key faculty people from the schools with which we were to work be present.

The parents and students arrived at the appointed hour. Their anger left no room for even a courteous introduction. Parent A spoke up as she entered the room: "I don't know what this meeting is all about. All we want is some police protection. We pay our taxes. Why are we speaking to you? This won't do any good, and besides we must be in church by 7 P.M. We've never missed a church meeting yet!" The rest of the group, not yet seated, jumped on the band-wagon.

Parent B: "I've made at least four or five calls to the Superintendent's office. Each time I'm connected to some stupid person in Community Relations who promises the Superintendent will phone me back. Have you ever spoken to him? Well, we can't get to him!"

I reflected a moment and said, "No. I was invited here by the Superintendent's Office, but I've never spoken to him directly."

Parent B: "Well, what are they calling you for? They're just passing the buck! Let them speak to us. We'll tell them what to do!"

Parent C: "Have you been to Central High? Have you seen all the Blacks congregate on the first floor and in front of the main entrance? No White kid can go through the front door. Why? Is that fair? Why do all the Blacks congregate on the front steps? The first floor is jammed with Blacks!"

I asked, "Where do the Whites congregate, on the second floor?"

Parent A screamed back, "Whites don't congregate! Sure they're on the second floor. They've got to be somewhere, but they don't congregate!" The message was emerging. When Blacks are together, they congregate. When Whites are together, they don't congregate. This was all said with grave sincerity. Prejudice does not lend itself to rational deduction.

Parent C: "Believe you me if the police were allowed in, the corridors would be cleared in two minutes."

Parent D: "Blacks should go back to Africa if they don't like it here. Whites are for Law and Order. We'll keep it that way!"

All of the parents were very involved in the discussion while their sons remained silent. These people's impotence to deal with the system was in contradiction to their praise for the establishment and their demand for law and order. When again they complained about the Administration going into hiding when a crisis occurred, I moved in: "People, I know the frustration you are experiencing in trying to work with our system. In Los Angeles I fought City Hall, even stood a five-week criminal trial as a defendant in order to get a single ordinance rescinded, an ordinance that made an innocent home-owner criminally liable if he could not repair the property damaged by a landslide. The developers and the building inspectors are exonerated, and the home-owner is doubly penalized for purchasing a home that the Department of Building and Safety had declared to be safe. Ten thousand homes and 39 lives have been lost, yet no one had fought City Hall. The ordinance was an open invitation to corruption between the developers and city officials. I won the criminal suit by a jury trial. The ordinance has at last been modified. It was not easy!"

I felt an immediate response by the entire group. They were all small home-owners. The possibility of losing their homes unjustly allowed them to identify with the problem. I continued: "If we cannot correct an inequity that should have been erased from the books in five minutes, how can we hope to rectify the major injustices in our society?"

There was a hushed silence. Finally, one boy began to speak, hesitatingly at first. "May I say something!"

His father moved in quickly: "Jim, you be quiet a minute! I want to say—"

I interrupted, "Just a minute, Mr. F. I'm interested in what your son has to say. I'll come back to you in a minute." The students, up to this point, had remained dramatically silent. They were the ones who had been injured and were entitled to be heard.

Jim continued: "Well, you know, I've been thinking! The Black kids are right to take over the front door. Look how many years they had to go through the back door! I can't really blame them for congregating at the front door now!"

I responded: "Jim, you're saying there's more to the problem than meets the eye."

Jim said, "Yeah! They never hurt anyone unless you ask for it."

Jim's dad quickly got into the act: "You didn't start it the day you were knocked unconscious, did you! Did you start it! Tell me!"

Jim said, "No, not really." I could feel him wince under his father's attack. This youngster was beginning to reevaluate the problem.

I said, "Jim, What really happened that day?"

Jim said, "Well, I was late to class so instead of using the side door, I used the front door, and the next thing I know, I was knocked unconscious."

I responded, "You're saying the incident could have been avoided."

Jim said, "Sure! It was like I was daring them!"

The other students now began to correct the distortions they had recounted to their parents. The parents kept quoting statements their sons had made, and the boys would say, "Yeah, but it wasn't exactly like that," or "Yeah, but you never listen to the whole story!"

One student added, "If the classes were better, we wouldn't be so bored. We've got to have some excitement at school!"

Parent D now spoke up. She had a plan all worked out for the solution of the problems. She referred to her notes: "One, the police should clear the corridors. Two, since most of the incidents occur during the lunch hour, there should be supervised games, pingpong tables, etc. with recreational workers planning the students' activities."

Her son was quick to speak up. "That costs money! How come you voted against the school tax?"

This completely took his mother off guard. "We shouldn't have to pay more taxes. The Superintendent doesn't do a damn thing. His salary could be used for this purpose. We should start a recall!"

Once more I moved in. "I agree that police who are armed could clear the corridors. The students are unarmed. The police, however, will never clear the feelings of injustice that are responsible for the problems. I hear, primarily, the blame-throwing: 'The Blacks cause the trouble'—'The police should be brought in'—'The Superintendent is at fault'—I heard only one boy say that perhaps he contributed to the problem."

Parent E interrupted: "Well, how come the Blacks never get hurt—just the Whites. Every day you read about another White kid being hurt at some school by a Black gang of thugs."

I said, "Perhaps Black students being injured won't make interesting news items."

The point hit hard. With amazement, she said, "Do you really mean Black kids are also hurt? They must be scared, too!"

I said, "Isn't it a pity that Black parents and White parents have to worry about the safety of their children when they send them to school?"

After a pause in which I could feel each member toy with a thought that had never occurred to them from their perspective, Jim spoke up. "You know each of us kids could do something. We raised lots of money for the March of Dimes. We also could begin to look at what we're doing that's messing us all up."

My faith in our youth is always bolstered by the Jims all over the country. I asked, "If I were able to arrange a meeting with the very Black kids that beat you up, would you fellows be willing to meet with them?"

The response in chorus was "Yes!" And Jim added, "It's about time we began to listen to each other."

Parent B brought the discussion back to the Superintendent and the Board. "If they can't be reached, nothing will ever be different!"

I responded, "I am going to meet with the Administrators tomorrow evening. Would you like me to set up an early appointment for you to meet with them?"

Parent D said: "You know, maybe we first should try to meet with the parents of the Black kids. If you say they are as worried as we are, maybe if we work together, we'll get something done."

All of the parents were eager to have this encounter, even though some of them admitted that they had never spoken to Blacks and would probably feel uncomfortable. They wondered whether the Blacks would be willing to talk to them. I agreed to explore the idea with the Black parents and arrange such a meeting if it were possible. These White parents were vaguely beginning to see how their racist attitudes were defeating their children's education.

The policeman glanced at his watch and commented that it was too late to attend the church meeting. Everyone laughed, and their cheerful departure was in great contrast to their hostile entrance.

The following day various prominent members of the community kept dropping in, offering opinions, particularly as to key people who would be offended if not contacted. We sorted out the relevant material that could be useful to our task and ignored the warnings of caution and futility. We, however, encouraged the community involvement at all times.

At 8 P.M. the administrative members and others began to arrive. The

Director of Counseling Services for the Department of Education was the only familiar face. He had observed a four-hour confrontation session I had conducted at Central High in 1968 because of racial tensions over the Martin Luther King Memorial Services. Consequently, when the Superintendent's Office requested my assistance in the current crisis, I had assumed that it was upon his recommendation since he was the only knowledgeable person on the staff who had observed my work. This erroneous assumption later presented embarrassing complications.

When the White counselor who had given Dawn such a rough time in Friday's session entered, he sought me out immediately. This time he made no attempt to conceal his hostility. His open anger was preferable to his contained rage. He said, "I saw you devastate two White boys. They left your session completely crushed! They will never be the same. I saw you devastate them!"

I responded, "I don't know much about them, but I must have devastated you."

He said, "Certainly, because of what you did to them. I'll make any wager they won't return to the group on Monday."

"What a pity," I said. "If they don't, they may miss an important opportunity. Tomorrow will tell the tale."

By 8:30 someone suggested that the meeting get underway. They had to be up early the next morning. I had been awaiting the Superintendent and Board Members, but then was told that the Superintendent was out of town, and the Board Members had not been invited.

"Oh!" I said. "The parents with whom I met yesterday are obviously correct. When a crisis occurs, everyone goes into hiding. Their concerns appear to be justified."

The Head of Public Relations was quick to speak up. "Who are these parents you referred to?"

I reviewed Saturday's session and stressed the complaints that the parents of the injured boys had made, their repeated phone calls to the Superintendent, the false promises that he would return the calls, and their feelings of impotence to get action.

Her response was simple: "We get the kookiest calls. Our Superintendent couldn't possibly waste his time returning them!"

I could not refrain from saying, "They may appear as kooky calls to you, but these people are hurting. They are worried about the safety of their children who have already been seriously injured. They are entitled to have direct contact with their Superintendent. What's more, it was so inconceivable to me that he would not want to meet with them that I told them I would set up such a meeting. They wish, however, to meet first with Black parents and then have their voices heard in unison. I am shocked that the Superintendent is not here this evening."

The Assistant Superintendent immediately accepted the responsibility of setting up a session with his superior and the Board Members for the following Friday evening, assuring me that in no way would this meeting with the parents be canceled.

The principal of South Junior High then shared his observation of the reduction in tension during the Friday sessions at his school. Concern was expressed that the program might be discontinued following our departure, primarily because of the reactionary Board Members. The vote among them was described as being $3\frac{1}{2}$ to $3\frac{1}{2}$. In other words, there were three ultraconservatives, three moderate liberals, and one unpredictable. We sensed the political arena that invariably precludes concern for real issues. Energy was centered on the power struggle among seven men, while education remained sterile. Without the backing of these seven men, our efforts would be futile. The buck stopped here. The responsibility for the violence rested with these seven men who politically could not agree with one another without forfeiting their party support. Their personal bias had barricaded the openness that dedication to education demands. We knew that our meeting with these gentlemen would be our most important challenge.

All through the discussion we were particularly aware of the principal of Hillside Junior High School despite his total silence. I finally said, "Mr H, you look troubled. Is there something you would like to say?"

He said, "When are you coming to Hillside? We need you there. There is hardly a day that we don't have some incident occur at our school. An explosion is imminent!" He was greatly relieved when Dr. Murillo agreed to go to his school the following day. We later learned that a plan to burn down that school during the Thanksgiving weekend was known to the police as well as to others. He remained after the meeting for a planning session with us.

The following morning when I returned to South, the principal announced several times over the public address system that only those students who had met with me on Friday were to go immediately to the teachers' cafeteria. Instead of the original twenty students, over a hundred youngsters responded to the announcement. I yelled above the noise: "Students, I'm delighted with your eagerness to participate in this problem-solving process. Unfortunately, I can't work with such a large group in this size room. I shall try to get to all of you, but I'm going to ask those who were not here Friday to return to your classes." About sixty of them left, and the remaining forty assisted in the arranging of chairs in a large circle. Once more, all the Blacks sat on one side and all the Whites on the other. We had each student pin on a name tag, and I wrote Zelda on mine. They were delighted that they could refer to me by my first name. We were now ready to begin our session. I noticed a change that had come over Rick, the angry White boy in Friday's encounter. He had a big smile and appeared relaxed. I said, "How are you, Rick?"

He seemed proud as he said, "I feel much better! I've done a lot of thinking, and I want to be friends, honest!" It was a spontaneous statement that left its impact upon the group. From the corner of my eye, I could see the White counselor wink at me and smile. He was a good sport in losing his wager.

Rick's opening remark brought a response from Don, the other student who had cried: "Me, too. I did lots of thinking! I wasn't scared to come to school today!"

I said, "Don, draw your chair into the center of the circle. How would you like to get to know one Black student?" He pulled his chair into the center and nodded his willingness. "Is there one Black student who would like to get to know Don?" I asked.

A Black boy pulled his chair along with him as he said, "Hi, Don." There was a silence, the clumsy embarrassment when two people don't know what to say to each other, and then these two boys began to explore the common denominator of human feelings. Their discovery of greater similarities than differences was deeply moving as they spoke of their feelings about their brothers and sisters, their loneliness, their poverty, their boredom in school, and their fear of failure. The future looked grim, particularly if they would have to go to war and get killed. The audience watched intently and came in touch with a new awareness as these two boys laid aside their anger and experimented with new ways of relating.

I used this moment of sensitivity to ask, "Is there ever any justification for a riot?"

There was a long pause followed finally by a Black girl saying, "Damn right!" Gloria was the smallest child in the group, frail and sad.

"Well, come into the center and tell us about it, Gloria," I said. "When do you feel riots are justified?"

She looked directly at the faculty standing together behind the circle and said, "When you're blamed for something you didn't do and no one will listen to you, no one will believe you—or when you did something bad, and you admit it, and they won't let you forget—they won't get off your back—Well, what else can you do?"

A White girl in the outer circle spoke up, "Oh! Excuse me! Oh, I owe you an apology! When you said that sometimes riots are all right, I hated you. I just hated you! And then I listened. I really listened and heard your reasons—and I feel the same way. I feel exactly the same way!"

And now these two girls were talking together, and Gloria was drying her tears with the back of her hand. A Black boy wiped his forehead and said, "Man! This is heavy!" I could see Martin Luther King patting the heads of these children who were joining hands to fight the injustices of the adult world surrounding them.

The children were dismissed for lunch only after exacting a promise from me that we would continue the following day.

When I arrived for Tuesday's session, the children had already arranged their own inner and outer circles and were involved in serious discussion about the changes needed in their school. The Blacks were again seated on one side and the Whites on the other. Their greeting of "Hi, Zelda" was a moment I shall never forget! I continued with their theme and suggested that they develop a planning session for necessary changes in education. They posted large sheets of paper on the wall and assigned the task to one student to write a list of items on which they all agreed.

1. No prejudiced teachers.
2. Old teachers have old ways—tenure can be bad.
3. Teachers can learn from students.
4. Teachers should respect students.
5. Students shouldn't be expelled for silly reasons.
6. Most of the rules should be changed.
7. Students should have a student lounge where they can go when classes are boring. No teachers!

At this point, a dramatic incident occurred. This school had a faculty lounge from which students were excluded. It was called "The Community Room." No sooner had point 7 been written down, than one of the Black leaders rose and said, "Hey kids! We've got a Community Room. We're members of the community. Let's take it over." The students got up, all 40 of them, and rushed toward the door. I knew I had to act quickly. I had been in the Community Room and knew there were seven or eight teachers in it. As loudly as I could, I said, "You've got a great idea, but you're going to defeat yourselves. Come back and let's first talk about it." The students returned to their respective places, the Blacks and Whites still separated. I said, "I think your idea is great. I can't promise you that you'll get your student lounge, but I know you won't get it this way. You said you want a lounge not supervised by teachers. I think teachers feel they must always be around because they see you as irresponsible—and I guess sometimes you act irresponsibly. Now might be the time for you to break up into four groups and develop a workable plan as to the furnishing and care of the lounge, the periods different classes may use it, the people to be in charge of it, etc."

The students spontaneously divided themselves into four groups with Blacks and Whites intermingled in each. Before the bell rang for lunch, they had posted on the wall a big sheet of paper on which was written in bold black letters: The next riot Blacks and Whites together.

A few minutes after the session had broken up, a teacher, ashen gray, rushed into the room and said, "Dr. Wolpe, did you tell the students to take over the Community Room? All 40 are in there!" I walked back to the lounge and had to refrain from laughing at the scene. Seven teachers were standing against the wall as if they had been lined up for a firing squad. They were so stiff it looked as if rigor mortis had set in. The students had helped themselves to cokes and coffee, had turned on the TV, and were sitting on the comfortable chairs as well as being sprawled over the floor. I said, very calmly, "Kids, are you telling me you don't want to work with me anymore?" With that simple question, the 40 students put down their coffee and cokes and left the Community Room. That day at lunch, for the first time in the history of the school, Blacks and Whites were seen eating together in the student cafeteria.

The afternoons were devoted to faculty sessions, the principal having arranged for 30 or more substitutes so that classes were not interrupted. Counselors from all of the schools were invited to participate. As I walked into the first meeting, I was struck by the division of color. The Blacks were in a corner, as far removed from the Whites as possible. Their angry comments were intended for my benefit:

"Another goddamn waste of time."
"I'm getting damn sick of sensitivity groups."
"I resent these meetings."
"They'll never know what it's all about."
"Nothing ever changes."

I walked into their huddle, and said: "I can't ask you to participate. You have expressed the futility of talking to Whites, but since I've come all the way from Los Angeles and don't want this to be a total waste, would you be willing to help me out? I would like to expose this white faculty to a training session in listening. I don't blame you for not wanting to talk to them, but would you mind getting into the center of the circle and talking among yourselves about your feelings or anything you would like to discuss? Don't talk to them. Just talk among yourselves and allow them to eavesdrop."

Jeanne, one of the most militant counselors, was the first to speak up. "Do you honestly think this will do any good? You know damn well they're never going to change!"

I responded, "I don't know what they're going to do. I'd settle for them just learning to listen. Besides, not too long ago, I was where they are now."

Another Black counselor said, "You were never there!"

And Jeanne added, "Right on!" Without too great reluctance they pulled their chairs into the center of the circle, and I addressed the White faculty.

"People, rarely do we listen. We have preconceived ideas and built-in pacifiers which allow us to defend ourselves and throw the blame on someone else. This is going to be a training session in listening. The people in the center are going to have a discussion among themselves. No one is to interrupt. You are only to listen."

The most poignant discussion unfolded as these 14 Blacks held up a mirror for Whites to reflect upon. They spoke of their impotence to get Whites to listen, of their hopelessness for change, of the Whites' inflexibility, of the American Dream that to them was a nightmare. They saw their own role primarily as helping Black students to get around the system. Something bad had to happen before Whites even gave lip-service to the problem, and then the solution was always further repressive tactics. They felt all Whites were responsible by default, and compared American society to Nazi Germany: "They're just like those Germans who closed their doors and drew their blinds and smelled the Jewish flesh burning. They allowed the Nazis to do what they did—Period! You know those Nazis could not have existed if they were not allowed to. The same thing applies to White racism, as far as I'm concerned!"

In response, another faculty member said, "So you're saying you want the White man to clean up his own house."

And a third member interrupted: "We can't clean his house. He won't even let us in. And how can we stand outside and sweep up the inside of his house? That's an impossible task—a waste of time!"

They spoke of how the same racist teachers who were messing up the minds of Black kids were also messing up the minds of White kids. "All education is messed up!" They pointed out how the rules of their educational system were racist. Black students were constantly being expelled, and Black kids on the streets rather than in school could never be helpful to anyone. They saw White teachers copping out by focusing their attention on discipline. "A good teacher doesn't have discipline problems!"

They spoke of how their school had been closed down for a few days in a previous uprising and workshops were instituted for the faculty. "We didn't accomplish one thing! The same teachers that were at the same meetings went back to their same classrooms and picked up where they left off the day before the school was closed!"

Another teacher added, "Tell us, tell us the correct dialogue that we should use with White people so that they will change their racist attitudes! We can't work with their hang-ups. They're sick to the core!"

When their dialogue ended, the Whites were asked to review what they had heard. Their defensiveness became offensive. One teacher stated: "We're thinking about our problems in the classroom, and last year I heard the figures mentioned that about 90% of our classroom discipline problems are Black students?" This teacher received much support from some of the other Whites. Another teacher stated that he had heard the Blacks speak only of White racism, and wondered about Black racism, a remark that brought immediate response from the Black group. "The definition in the dictionary is the assumption of superiority by one race over another and the discriminatory practices thereof! And Black people have not perpetuated nor perpetrated any such situation on White people!"

It was at this point that I asked: "Why would it have been better if the Blacks had spoken of Black racism? What would that have done for you?" This was a turning point in the discussion that led to self-examination, from the denial of prejudice by the Whites to the discovery of their biases and major responsibility for the existent problems. A White teacher responded to my question: "Damn it! We're throwing blame again! We've watched this happening and we've not done anything but call the Black kids thugs! We know damn well if we were really educators none of this could happen! It's about time we began to take some risks, even if we have to be fired. All we do is expel the Black kids! That's not education!"

The White faculty began the painful soul-searching process, and the Blacks began to relax. The tension lifted as together they moved into a planning session for changes in education. They recognized the boredom in many of their classes, the racist rules that they were abiding by, the poor textbooks that they detested using. On and on they went with their dissatisfactions and lack of enthusiasm in their professional lives. By the end of the third session, Jeanne, who had been so resistant initially to the meeting, initiated a petition directed to the Board members, requesting an on-going program in human relations. This petition was signed by 100 Black and White faculty members. The students also filed a petition with 500 signatures, which they presented to the Board following our departure.

Because we had received no official confirmation of the Parent–Administration meeting for Friday, I announced at the close of the last faculty meeting that we would be returning to Los Angeles on Thursday, Thanksgiving Day. I suspected my message would be relayed to the Superintendent, and that evening he phoned to invite Dr. Murillo and me to lunch on Friday. My response was, "Are you saying that the meeting with the parents and the Board is not to take place Friday evening!"

"Oh!" he said, "This is the Thanksgiving weekend. I have irreversible plans!"

I responded, "We will return to Los Angeles tomorrow. We don't wish to be here for the explosion!"

Needless to say, he discovered his plans were alterable and promised that all the Board Members would be present. He realized that he had better be briefed on what had been occurring during the week and spent all day Friday in conference with us. He was concerned that Blacks and Whites would be present at the meeting and wanted the assurance that there would be no outbreak of violence. I could only assure him that there would be a far greater possibility of violence if such a meeting did not take place.

Prior to the Board meeting, the Black and White parents, accompanied by their children, worked jointly on their grievances and strategy for the presentation. The Board Members were not to commit themselves to false promises but were to reevaluate their responsibility for the current crisis. This session was the dramatic highlight of the week. Both parents and students actively participated in a four-hour session, never once losing the issue. The Board asked for the weekend to consider the grievances and said that they would report back at a special open meeting the following Monday evening.

Realizing the importance of working with the attitudes of the seven Board members, I suggested to the Superintendent that he arrange a cocktail party for an informal sharing of our concerns. The following morning his call confirming the get-together interrupted our conference with the editor of the *Gazette*. I was furious when I returned from the phone because my son and daughter-in-law had not been included. The editor quietly asked, "Who phoned you to come out here?"

I replied, "We came at the request of the Superintendent."

He said, "I didn't ask that? Who specifically phoned you?"

I never understood more clearly the meaning of Karl Buhler's, "Ah Ha!" response. The Superintendent had found it difficult to say "No" to my son. No one had ever really approved of our presence. The following night at the cocktail party I presented the following statement to the seven Board Members and the 100 invited guests:

"I ask that you drink a toast to your two uninvited guests. I have made a terrible error which I must now attempt to rectify. I moved into your community because I had made a false assumption. Two years ago I had had the privilege of meeting the Chief of Counseling for your educational system. He had come to my son's home to discuss the racial tensions at Central High School. At that time we set up a session for the Administration, Heads of Departments, and others, and we resolved the crisis. Therefore, when my son phoned me ten days ago and stated that the Superintendent's office had officially sanctioned Dr. Murillo's and my services to deal with the racial problem, I had assumed that this had occurred on this gentleman's suggestion. He was the only member of the Administration who had observed my work and was qualified to make such a recommendation.

"As our week progressed, I became increasingly critical of this community. Never in our experience had we been forced to work against such resistance when we had been invited to assist in a community problem. It was not until yesterday that I could get off the blame-throwing trip of mine and begin some self-examination:

1. A whole community could not be wrong.
2. Why had people who invited us gone into hiding?
3. Were we the only ones aware of the crisis, while everyone else was able to enjoy the Thanksgiving Holiday?
4. Who had invited us?

"A flash of blinding light! My son! He had always had an exaggerated confidence in my ability and a dedicated concern for the welfare of children. It was he who had stuffed us down your throat! We were truly the unwanted guests, presumptuous to know what was good for your community. You had never wanted what was perceived as sensitivity training in the first place. All along I was blaming you for not welcoming guests who had been thrust at you; even worse, guests for whom you felt compelled to pay a high fee for services you did not even know whether or not you wanted. How pompous we must have appeared to you because of my false assumption!

"Dr. Murillo and I discussed our learning experience together, laughed at my error that had so boxed us into a ridiculously difficult situation, and decided that whether you wanted it or not, you at least have had a *free* sample of what our approach to community problem-solving is all about. We ask that you try to forget that we entered your community and review again your own approaches to problem-solving. You might now want to experiment with police protection or any other program as you search for your solution. If at any time your Board unanimously decides that they might find it helpful to consult with us and extends an invitation to us, we will do all possible to return to your community. Again, I ask your forgiveness for having imposed our methods on your community. Yet I cannot be too regretful for I have learned from my error and hope to become a better community consultant because of it. Tomorrow we leave for Los Angeles."

Lively discussion followed this toast. The immediate reaction was one of fear, which we capitalized upon by assuring them of the likelihood of further explosive incidents if changes were not instigated. At the same time, we let them know that the current crisis was sufficiently resolved for us to leave without too grave concern, provided they acted quickly in reviewing the grievances. When asked why my return demanded a unanimous decision of the Board rather than a simple majority, my response was: "If we can't get seven men together on this most serious issue, how can we hope to get the community together?" One of the most conservative members of the Board began his statement with, "As to these sensitivity groups, maybe it's my ignorance, but..." I interrupted with, "That's right!" The laugh broke the tension and allowed me to say, "We could have been brainwashing your children's minds all week, yet none of you came to see what was happening! The sessions were open to everyone!" For three hours, the discussion continued as they laid the foundation for new directions.

The results of psychologists working with this community were:

1. The police were not brought into the schools.
2. Human relation programs were substituted for the police.
3. The *Gazette* continued its articles regarding the problems in the school system for months following our visit.
4. Many of the racist rules were dropped.
5. Teachers, regardless of tenure, were dismissed if shown to be overtly racist, whereas previously they were transferred to other schools.

6. When compulsory busing was later introduced, the only three schools that did not experience a single racial incident were the three schools with which we had worked.

7. I was invited to return to set up further workshops in human relations, which implied the unanimous decision of the Board members. (My hospitalization prevented my acceptance, and consultants from the State University were used for the on-going program.)

In this case presentation two psychologists were able to bring about some social awareness that has left its impact upon the community. It is to be emphasized that more often than not when a consultant is called into a community for crisis intervention the establishment desires the cessation of violence without the change of the status quo of the system. There is always, therefore, the danger of further embedding and perpetuating the racism once the crisis has been terminated. The aim must be the resolution of the nuclear conflicts responsible for the crisis in the first place. Corrective measures demand continuous organized and vigilant community involvement. Men committed to education must encourage this or be removed from office. White racism and outworn educational procedures within our system are responsible for the uprisings. The men in power can be forced to deal with these problems by community action and cooperative working together. Otherwise, we will move from crisis to crisis.

The following case presentation is more impressive because the entire community of psychologists in Los Angeles mobilized its resources and succeeded in bringing about significant social change in the County and City of Los Angeles. Its impact has been felt across the country, with many states now reevaluating their Civil Service procedures.

RECTIFYING THE INEQUITIES BEHIND CIVIL SERVICE EXAMINATIONS

On September 2, 1969, elimination of all racial barriers in hiring and promotions of County employees was ordered by the Los Angeles Board of Supervisors. The unanimous action of the Board was hailed as a milestone in dealing with racial embeddedness. The County Personnel Director was instructed to make a progress report in three months and additional reports every six months thereafter. At that time, there were ten Blacks in the department of over 1800 firemen. The Fire Department specifically was directed to recruit minorities for the Civil Service Examination to be held in 1971.

The County Fire Fighters' Union elicited the enthusiastic response of approximately 2000 qualified Blacks and Chicanos when told that they would be given a racially unbiased examination and would be welcomed as employees in the Fire Department.

A month prior to filing for the examination, however, the recruits learned of the Personnel Department's intention to hold a "random selection" or lottery, limited to only 500 who would be permitted to take the Civil Service Examination. The Department attributed the necessity for such a procedure to its insufficient personnel for the administration of the oral examination. It was then that I was approached by some of our Black citizens to intercede. I attended a meeting scheduled by the Chief of Employment for the L.A. County Personnel Department, who initiated the conference by stating that he understood we were opposed to the random selection procedure and wished to enlighten us as to its merit. He went on to say that in the first training class for new firemen they would have 12 Blacks, 12 Chicanos, and 12 Whites. I interrupted by saying, "Are you now doing selective hiring?"

He became obviously embarrassed by the question and said that they hoped to get that percentage from the random selection, a puzzling statement in view of the fact that they expected twice as many Whites filing for the examination but would have two-thirds of the first slots filled by minorities. He spoke of their sincere commitment to the Affirmative Action Program and, in view of their recognition of their previously racially biased written examination, they had now decided to base the competitive grade solely on the oral examination. In the past, however, even if a candidate scored 100% on the written and 69% on the oral he was failed. In effect, selective hiring had always been used in the name of Civil Service. This procedure undoubtedly accounted for the exclusion of minorities. When questioned about the objectivity of the oral examiners, his response was that Blacks do better on an oral than on a written examination. I pointed out that they could not have done so well on the oral in view of the fact that there were only nine Blacks out of 2000 hired. We were more interested in how many minorities had passed the written but failed the oral. Those figures were not made available to us.

We then referred to the County Charter section specific to open Civil Service Examinations which, in effect, stated that all qualified citizens must be permitted to take such an examination. He then proceeded to show us a letter from the County attorney, which stated that in his opinion if the case were brought to court he could undoubtedly win it because there was no alternative solution to their personnel problem. When asked how many vacancies would occur during the year, the response was somewhere between 180 and 200. He refused, however, to commit himself to proportionate hiring of 60-60-60 as he had indicated in the first group of 12-12-12. I shared with him my fantasy. I had visions of the headlines in the *Los Angeles Times*: "Two-Thirds Minorities Hired in Los Angeles County Fire Department." The director and chief of personnel would look as if they had done a good job, but I was personally unimpressed by such tokenism. The oral examination from here on out could be used to further exclude minorities and perpetuate the racism. I finally said, "Mr. Marcus, we won't let you do this. We will bring this before the community through all of the news media. We will fight this in court. You have had two years to rectify this problem and, if this is the best you could come up with, something must be done."

I further pointed out that they had done active recruitment, given hope to 2000 minorities and now wouldn't even permit 87% of them to take the examination. Such hopelessness for change is the impetus for violence, and the men in power must be held responsible when it occurs. Another reminder that the press release would go out that day made Mr. Marcus obviously uncomfortable. He asked for an extension of time. In a week he might hit upon a different solution. Another conference was set up for the following week.

Knowing the County Attorney's argument in the event of a law suit, we had to produce alternative solutions to their personnel problem. The oral examination in particular concerned us, especially since they had no minorities on their Examining Boards. The Personnel Chief had already informed us that though they were forbidden to put the ethnic origin on the application blank, the Personnel Department had secretly coded each applicant when he filed for the examination. Regardless of how biased the written examination was, there was no criteria whatsoever for grading the oral examination. Our first proposal, therefore, at the next meeting was that everyone be given the same written examination, but that they select their employees from the upper 10% of each ethnic group. The minorities would thereby be competing among themselves rather than against the Whites. This far more equitable solution was totally nonacceptable to Mr. Marcus. His rationale for turning down this suggestion was that he would be unable to get the Civil Service Commissioners, men supposedly committed to fair examinations for all, to understand converted scores.

Our next proposal was more difficult for Mr. Marcus to reject. He had repeatedly stated that he would prefer having everyone take the examination, but their insufficient number of oral examiners made this an impossible task. When asked the qualifications for an oral examiner, he stated, "You have to have a Bachelor's degree from a good University and understand motivation."

I immediately replied, "We'll do better! I will guarantee you 100 or more Ph.D. psychologists or M.D. psychiatrists who have devoted much of their life-study to motivation. We will give you as many examiners as you require for administering the oral examinations. We will even have minorities on our Boards, and we won't charge the County one cent for our services. You, however, will have to give us your criteria for grading the examination. This will permit everyone who qualifies to take it."

I also asked him his definition of motivation. His response was unbelievable: "Oh," he said, "If you ask a man why he wants to be a fireman and he says because he needs the money, well, obviously that is poor motivation."

I responded, "Mr. Marcus, you fail them for being honest? If they told me they enjoyed putting out fires, I might worry about them!" I then learned that never have they had a standardization or validation of the examinations they had until now been using. Not until that moment did I appreciate my naivete regarding Civil Service Examinations.

My offer had pulled the rug from under the Chief. He could find no flaw in our proposal. He asked that we put it in writing, and he would recommend its acceptance to the Director of Personnel. I knew I had committed my colleagues without even getting their permission, yet I hadn't the slightest anxiety regarding their support. We had 24 hours in which to submit the following proposal:

September 18, 1971

Mr. Elliot Marcus
Chief, Employee Selection Division
Department of Personnel, Los Angeles County

Dear Mr. Marcus:

We are submitting to you our formalized proposal that will allow *all* candidates who file for the Civil Service Examination for the Fire Department to take it. Our proposal eliminates the possibility of serious repercussions from all members who had been actively recruited only to later be disallowed such opportunity to compete in the examination because of your proposed random selection of 500 candidates.

We recognize that such random selection proposals stemmed from your inadequate budget that does not allow for the sufficient staffing necessary to administer 5,000 or more oral examinations.

To avoid the possibility of crises, law suits and further inequities, we propose for this current emergency the following:

1. We will provide an ample number of trained, qualified Ph.D. psychologists and M.D. psychiatrists to conduct the oral examinations on a volunteer basis.
2. The number of professionals will be determined by the number of candidates who file for the examination October 16, 1971.
3. Each interviewer will submit to you a vita indicating his background and qualifications.
4. You will have the privilege of screening the examiners for your approval.
5. You will submit to the examiners the criteria for grading the candidates.
6. You will conduct one or more training sessions for the examiners, acquainting them with every aspect of the Department's needs that could be important in making the determinations by the examiners.
7. You will notify us in writing no later than the fourth of October your acceptance or rejection of this proposal along with Mr. Nesvig's official commitment.

We wish to emphasize that this is solely a stop-gap emergency procedure. We trust that by the next examination you will resolve your internal problems so that inequities are eliminated.

Respectfully submitted,

Seven days later we received the following response:

County of Los Angeles
Office of the Director of Personnel

September 24, 1971
Dear Dr. Wolpe:

Thank you for your proposal on the upcoming Firemen examination. There is a good deal of merit in the proposal and, if it were possible, I would endorse such a procedure. However, in all candor, I must admit that I am skeptical of your ability to produce the 700 man days necessary to interview 5,000 candidates. Further, I am sure you realize that 5,000 is only an estimate of the minimum filing we anticipate; and, in fact, the filing may well exceed that.

In light of this, I am instructing my staff to continue their preparation of the examination as it is currently proposed, i.e., use random selection to limit the number of candidates participating in the examination to 500. If, however, you can show reliable evidence of your ability to produce the required number of interviews, I am quite willing to consider a new examination format.

Again, thank you for your efforts and interest in seeing the County's Affirmative Action Program work.

Sincerely,
Gordon T. Nesvig, Director of Personnel

My response was brief:

Dear Mr. Nesvig:

I can hardly blame you for your skepticism of my ability to produce the number of man days required to interview the candidates. That is solely because you do not know me or my colleagues. I will have the hours pledged along with the vitas in your office by October 12th. We are also eliciting the assistance of the communication media to bring this to the attention of the community. If it is imperative that you have the list of volunteers in your office prior to October 12th or if you still have resistance to our proposal, we will be happy to meet with you personally to resolve our differences.

Most sincerely,

The fight was now on. That night 1500 letters to psychiatrists and 500 letters to psychologists were printed and ready for mailing the following day. The following is a copy of the letter:

September 25th, 1971

Dear Colleague:

Ninety-nine and one-half per cent of firemen in the Los Angeles County Fire Department are Whites. Because of the County's Affirmative Action Program, the Department was given two years to rectify this racial imbalance. The Fire Department Union did intensive recruiting and elicited the enthusiasm of 2,000 qualified Minority people to file on October 6, 1971, for a fair Civil Service Examination to be given at a future date.

Now the Department has no staff to administer the oral examination on which the competitive grade-rating is determined since the written examination is on a pass-fail basis. Despite the fact that the law specifically states that *all qualified people* are entitled to take the examination, the solution to their staff problem is to have a random selection in which only the first 500 names pulled from the pool of 4,000 Whites and 2,000 Minorities will be permitted to take the examination. This obviously does not insure the most qualified people to take the examination. It rather insures the further distrust of the Minorities who had been actively recruited to take the examination.

Because of this deplorable perpetuation of injustice in the name of Civil Service, we submitted the enclosed proposal. Also enclosed is the County's response to our proposal.

If we band together, dedicated to rectify this blatant injustice by volunteering our time to administer the oral examinations, we can accomplish the following:

1. All future examinations must be standardized on a population including Minorities.
2. The examination must correlate with job performance. In the past the level of reading was the primary determinant for passing the test and excluding Minorities.
3. All qualified people regardless of race will have a fair chance on the examination.
4. Los Angeles could be the model that demonstrates to our Society how professionals can use their professional skill and training to eliminate the inequities in our system.

The emergency is grave. If the County is allowed to follow through on their procedure, they will set a precedent that will further perpetuate rather than eliminate racism.

Please sign the enclosed form together with your vita and commit yourself to a minimum of four to eight hours a week for three weeks so that we may get the task accomplished.

Most sincerely,

This letter was mailed September 25th. By September 30th we had over 4000 hours committed, 54 hours by psychiatrists, 270 hours by social workers, and over 3700 hours by psychologists whose vitas were more impressive than the Who's Who around the world. Along with this most generous response, I received the following two endorsements:

The Board of Directors of the Los Angeles County Psychological Association by unanimous vote on October 21, 1971, extends their full support for your efforts to develop a more reliable examination in order to make County Civil Service more equitable to all applicants.

Sincerely,
Martin Reiser, Ph.D.
President

The Psychological Center of Los Angeles, the community service arm of the psychological professional association, enthusiastically endorses the program initiated by psychologists that would allow every eligible person who filed for the October 16th Civil Service Examination to be allowed to take it. The County of Los Angeles, despite insufficient staff, must meet the commitment it has made to the Affirmative Action Program in order to end the racial imbalance in employment. To test only a random selection of 10% of those qualified will not assure an increase in minority hires. The Psychological Center volunteers to assist in any way possible in the administration of these examinations to assure an equal opportunity to all qualified applicants. We shall be looking forward to active participation with you.

Sincerely,
Marvin Spanner, Ph.D.
President

Fortified by my colleagues' committed hours and the unequivocal support of our psychological associations, we instituted a citizen's action suit against the County of Los Angeles. The judge issued a temporary injunction barring the random selection. Later he reversed his decision, but the injunction held pending our appeal, which we won in October 1972.

In the interim, the following letter was sent to Senator Allan Cranston, the Civil Rights Commission, the Department of Labor, the A.C.L.U., etc.

November 18, 1971

Senator Allan Cranston
The United States Senate
Washington, D.C.

Dear Senator Cranston:

When recently the Los Angeles County's Department of Personnel announced its intention to hold a random selection limited to only 500 out of the 3600 qualified applicants who had filed for the upcoming Civil Service Examination for Fireman, I was approached by some of our Black citizens to intercede on their behalf. In investigating past policy in order to evaluate the current recommendations for change, I quickly discovered that more serious than the problem of random selection was the myth of Civil Service Examinations and the many inequities that have always been hidden behind the Civil Service label. I will attempt to outline the main problems uncovered that demand an investigation of our entire Civil Service process.

1. Selective Hiring:

Selective hiring rather than Civil Service has always, in effect, been the policy. Past examinations forced the exclusion of Minorities. The recognition of the unfairness of the written examination was admitted to by Elliott Marcus, Chief of the Employment Division of the Los Angeles County. In the past the cut-off point for the written examination was at the 90th percentile, thus allowing only 10% of applicants to pass. In addition, if an applicant scored 100% on his written examination, but failed the oral, he automatically was failed. The oral examiner thus had the power to disqualify any applicant regardless of his written examination score. The end result is that $99\frac{1}{2}\%$ of County firemen are currently White.

2. Subjective Evaluation:

To rectify this deplorable situation, the County has decided to lower the cut-off point to the 10th percentile for the written examination. Instead of a grade, however, they would be scored pass-fail and the entire competitive grade determination would now be based on the oral examination. When questioned regarding the subjectivity of the oral examiners, Mr. Marcus claimed that Minorities do better on an oral than on a written examination. He could not state the basis for his belief nor would he give us the figures as to how many Minorities had passed the written but failed the oral examination. The fact remains that only $\frac{1}{2}\%$ of the firemen in the L.A. County Fire Department are Blacks (9 out of 2000 firemen are Black).

3. Non-Standardization of Examinations:

Neither the oral nor written examinations have ever been standardized, correlated with job performance, or had determinations made of their reliability or validity. A Ph.D. psychologist in the Los Angeles County Personnel Department informed me that for the past ten years or more she has unsuccessfully urged the standardization of Civil Service examinations, but has been denied permission by their Chief.

By placing the competitive score solely on the subjective whim of the examiner in the attempt to rectify a long-standing injustice, and because an Affirmative

Action commitment was demanded, is to go from a bad situation to a worse one. They could have validated a test in the two years they have had to rectify the problem and, had they used Minorities in the standardization process, they could have come up with a reasonably fair test. Now they have set a precedent that officially perpetuates Selective Hiring in the name of Civil Service.

4. The Farce of Recruitment:

As part of the Affirmative Action Program, the Fire Department Union was directed to recruit Minorities, and they were successful in eliciting an enthusiastic response from 2000 Minorities who qualified to file for the examination. The active recruitment was obviously a waste of tax-payers' money. Having switched from a written grade to an oral grade, the County did not take into consideration the need for increased personnel to administer the orals to the increased number of applicants. In order to deal with this problem the Personnel Director ordered a random selection procedure that would limit the taking of the examination to only 10% of the candidates who had been actively recruited. The results of such random selection are:

A. No guarantee that the most qualified will even be permitted to take the examination. This negates the whole theory behind Civil Service and is in opposition to our charter.
B. No guarantee that the racial imbalance will be rectified by this procedure.
C. Now pressure is on to hire Minorities. What happens when the pressure is off? This could be the tokenism that allows the perpetuation of racism in our establishment.

5. No Rationale for Criteria for Oral Examinations:

Though the City Charter, the Federal Constitution and our state laws require all qualified citizens be permitted to take an open Civil Service examination, the County Personnel Director insisted that there was no alternative to their decision of random selection because of their staff shortage. I, therefore, suggested that psychologists, whose academic training and experience far exceeds their requirements for oral examiners, be permitted to volunteer their services for the administration of the examination without cost to the County. All we asked in return was that the County give us their criteria for grading the examination since a precise grading is mandatory on a competitive examination. Our proposal was turned down despite the fact that we had sufficient hours committed by psychologists to examine 10,000 candidates. Less than 3600 candidates filed for the examination. The County's insistence upon their solution is in opposition to its plea for community involvement by our citizens. Such denial breeds an expression of hopelessness by the recipients of the inequities; yet when violence occurs because of such hopelessness, we are told that we can work with our system.

6. Civil Service Hearing:

On October 26, 1971, we brought the matter to the Superior Court, and, among other charges, we pointed out that the requirement that adoption and amendment of Commission Rules be made only after Public Notice and Hearing had not been complied with. The Civil Service Commission, therefore, held an open hearing on

November 10, 1971, an open hearing wherein the decision had obviously been made behind closed doors. Though hundreds of citizens had given up their valuable time to protest the Commission's proposal with convincing arguments, the Commission unanimously voted in favor of random selection. Such deafness to citizens, dedicated to rectify injustice, can only further the disenchantment with our government. The myth of Democracy becomes increasingly more apparent. Our Court Hearing is scheduled for November 29, 1971.

It does not seem to matter who gets into office. The inequities continue, and the voice of the people is ignored. If you have any suggestions as to how we can work with our system, I would greatly appreciate your help.

Sincerely yours,

Response was immediate. Allan Cranston's Aide in Washington, D.C., phoned to say that Senator Cranston was now initiating a complete investigation of all Civil Service in the State of California. The Civil Rights Commission phoned to say that a bill was just passed that permitted the Federal Government to take action against a state, city, or county when racial discriminatory practices were in evidence. The Justice Department phoned to say that because of the psychologists' groundwork, Los Angeles would be the first city to be investigated under the new law. Three attorneys from the U.S. Justice Department came to Los Angeles to discuss the case with us and to initiate their investigation.

The Justice Department chose to file against the City of Los Angeles rather than the County, a decision difficult to comprehend in view of the fact that though the City also has demonstrated severe discriminatory practices in their Fire Department, it is not nearly as bad as that within the County.

A spark of light in an abysmal arena must intensify rather than diminish our efforts. We must never relax our vigilance. The establishment excels in double talk. On December 27, 1972, an attorney from the Justice Department phoned to inform me that the City was requesting a dismissal of the case against it, but he assured me that with relative certainty he would be able to prevent such dismissal. He then inquired about the disposition of the case against the County. I reviewed for him our success in winning the appeal and that to date the County has been unable to hire any firemen unless oral examinations are administered to all candidates. My delight in our success was not shared by him; rather, he recommended that we immediately contact an attorney currently in private practice but who was formerly with the Justice Department and completely familiar with the facts. The urgency in his suggestion was my impetus for immediate action, and I set up an appointment with the attorney for the following day. Just prior to my leaving for his office, I learned that the County was pulling one more of its shenanigans. It had called the top 500 candidates who had passed the written examination, which was never intended to be used as a competitive differentiation, for their oral interviews and was planning to make their official lists for hiring. There were only 13 Blacks in that top 500 which, if all had been hired, would have brought the percentage of Blacks from $\frac{1}{2}$% to 1%, and would have frozen the list for another two years. We had five days in which to get a temporary injunction and prevent the County's unfair procedure. A new case was filed in the Federal Court, the injunction was granted, and the hearing before Judge Gray took place on June 5th, 6th, and 7th at which time Judge Gray ordered 40% minorities in all future hiring be mandatory.

Despite the fact that this might be looked upon as an important step in the direction of removing racial discriminatory practices in governmental hiring, the 40% figure was a grave disappointment to us and indicates how even our judicial system demands the on-going patience of minorities. The judge went so far as to say that in issuing his order he was cognizant that Whites would be penalized, that in effect he was now dealing with reverse discrimination, but he saw no alternative. Such insensitivity to the suffering we have imposed upon minorities for hundreds of years and the concern about reverse discrimination when the shoe is not even on the toe of the other foot reflects the deep embeddedness of racism in our system. The term of "Reverse Discrimination" is synonymous with maintaining the status quo. The following article, published in the *Los Angeles Sentinel* and in *The Canyon Crier*, reflects my views:

"Reverse Discrimination"
by Zelda Wolpe

When the shoe is on the other foot and pinches, the scream of "Reverse Discrimination" blasts out. Such a slogan is, in reality, a plea for maintaining the status quo. No one for the past fifty years was too concerned with the discriminatory practices in the Los Angeles County Fire Department against Minorities, yet when the Federal Court Case against the County for just such practices was concluded June 7, 1973, Judge Gray was apologetic because some Whites might be penalized by his Court Order that demands 20% Blacks and 20% Chicanos be included in future hiring until respective percentage of community Minorities is attained. Such apology to Whites is hardly appropriate when currently over 97% of the firemen are still White. With only 100 firemen a year being hired it will take over fourteen years to reach an equitable balance, even using Judge Gray's erroneous figures. (There are 14% rather than his figure of 11% Blacks in our community, and 2100 firemen in the L.A. County rather than 1800.)

Unless Whites are willing to give up something, namely their monopoly of 97% of desirable positions, we will constantly struggle with ghettos, racial tensions, crime and racism. We can have no mental health or genuine education when prejudice and greed permeate our society. Judge Gray's decision was minimal token-ism to rectify this inequity. The Minorities will have to wait another fourteen years before an approximation of proportionate hiring is accomplished.

In summary, it is hoped that these case presentations might be the impetus for psychologists to reevaluate their responsibility in community involvement. Each of us has untapped resources that could eradicate White racism in our society. We Can Fight City Hall must be our commit-ted slogan.

Part V

An Overview

CHAPTER 12

Summary and Conclusions

No SINGLE book could encompass all the important or useful information about mental health and the urban poor. The existing perspectives on theory, training, practice, and research have been evolving over recent decades but have yet to reach the stage of coherency. Mental health workers around the country practice in their own ways, dealing with their own problems with poor clientele from their own perspectives; generally, they have little input into those corridors of power where policy decisions occur that ultimately impact upon practice. Despite the personal insights developed by the workers in the field, few people ever manage to have their knowledge utilized in the formation of training models or in drafting legislation setting mental health policy.

Workers are a part of the zeitgeist and are themselves the results of it. It is the popularly accepted beliefs and stereotypes persisting from historical myths about the urban poor, the mentally ill, and the value of the mental health worker that determine the support, encouragement, and opportunity provided the worker. The message so far has been inconsistent and ambivalent; the future directions remain vague. In the remaining few pages we shall review some of the factors that are important in understanding mental health problems of the urban poor.

The struggle for mental health is with us all. We carry signs of our successes by our demonstrations of personal competence, happiness, and perspective. We show our failures in our psychopathological symptoms, our lack of integration, our unhappiness, and our incompetence. Billingsley makes clear that the struggle is in all of us, but that little national attention is focused on our common needs. Mastery of life and concomitant mental health results from a confluence of forces, those within ourselves and those that make up the fabric of society. The poor are the "victims" of birth, inheritance, ignorance, and all the forces of subtle and obvious nature that conspire to perpetuate incompetence. The development of symptoms (or defects in mental health) represents the ultimate display of diminished ability to manage against the contingencies of life, i.e., to find a competent pattern of behavior. The mental "illness" of the poor is inherently no different than the illness of the rich; the differences lie in the contingencies of life, which often differ dramatically. The poor are often without recourse, without available resources to develop conventionally defined competencies, and without the protections from reality demands that are available to the affluent. Many of the survival skills learned by poor people are unfamiliar and unnecessary to the rich. These survival skills go unrecognized or may even be labeled as pathological. A middle-class mental health worker may see his poor client as devoid of resources and skills because the perspectives on life and personal priority differ between the two. As with conversations between people of differing native languages, the level of understanding and empathy is distorted by ignorance attributable to the failure of each to know the language of the other.

The poor have problems in living parallel to but different from those of the mental health professional. By virtue of having little money, they have not been active consumers in the fee-for-service mental health industry. They have not often significantly contributed to the training of mental health professionals or the shaping of attitudes and values of the developing leadership of the mental health professions. The orthodox psychoanalytic tradition, which has so strongly influenced mental health practice in this country, was constructed from experience with clients of middle-class values and did not need to incorporate the reality problem of survival often pressing on the poor, would-be client.

Why have the would-be poor clients not become actual clients? The mental health establishment has not "treated" the poor with much interest because of negative beliefs and values. Included are the attitudes held by many that the techniques of psychotherapy were not likely to be successful with the poor; the worker's feeling of impotence when confronted with the client's myriad of reality concerns, presumed and real pathology; the prejudice against the habits, race, language, or values of the poor client; the lack of financial and personal-social rewards in treating the poor client; and the blindness to alternative technique and resource inculcated by the training of the mental health establishment. Many of these "attitude problems" are dealt with by authors in this book. Lerner talks of the bias and prejudice that have prevented the mental health professions from trying to utilize their skills in a democratic way to face the issues of conflict in value or preference. Goldberg and Kane describe a direct approach to the lack of symmetry and respect for values in their search for equity and the provision of "services in-kind." Ranz and Dunn suggest that the model in use throughout the country for training psychiatrists is partly responsible for the small numbers of psychiatrists ending up in service with the poor. Following Riessman's analysis, it is easy to understand that despite the elegant words and intentions the disappointing lack of achievements in mental health can be traced to poorly articulated goals and the failure to develop strategies to meet them.

The poor are victims of many of the same problems ascribed to the mental health professions. The poor have not sought out or demanded mental health services; they have not lobbied for effective social legislation, picketed outrageous clinics, or participated in advisory bodies designed to develop mental health care delivery programs. Why? Probably many poor subscribe to the same prejudices and biases held by the mental health establishment. Their definition of the available resources, their own pattern of labeling symptoms, and their fear of "the man" have all contributed to the otherwise paradoxical lack of demand for mental health services from the poor. Change will need to come jointly from all involved.

As mentioned above, one of the "arguments" offered by mental health professionals for avoiding actively working with the poor is that the standard armamentarium of the mental health professional is not effective with the poor client. Lerner argues persuasively in her chapter and elsewhere that, at best, this is an untested prejudgment and represents resistance of the therapist. It seems likely that the professional does not find many personal rewards or satisfaction (as well as monetary gain) from working with the poor. Many professionals do not like poor people, devalue the poor's life-style, and subscribe to myths about the poor's lack of civilized values, inadequate motivation, and inability to comprehend. Unchallenged and unrecognized prejudice is likely to destroy a therapeutic relationship and in so doing confirm the expectations for failure on both sides. The separation is mutually reinforcing.

On the simplest level, language use differences could be expected to have an impact on the nature of insight derived from the therapeutic process. If the client suffers from "nerves," implying some biological dysfunction, the therapist may feel at a loss to translate this for the client into the metaphor of psychodynamics. Confronted with the seeming impossibility of insight, the next step is usually "supportive therapy"—all too often an euphemism for therapeutic inaction. Certain techniques suited to middle-class patients may be inappropriate for the poor client; however, the majority of problem-solving, analytical, and skill-developing tasks are suited to the poor and need only be translated to the reality of the poor client's experience. This can be accomplished with diligence by a sensitive clinician, or may be more easily achieved through the use of adjunct help—the indigenous paraprofessional. (Some of the problems of using the paraprofessional without clarifying role distinctions and expectations can be found in the work of Riessman.)

Goldstein (1973) discusses in detail the specifics of effective and ineffective therapeutic strategies with the poor. Following an extensive review of the research bearing on producing change in the poor client, Goldstein presents his suggestions for a systematic therapy. "Structured Learning Therapy" per Goldstein is a combination of modeling, role-playing, and judicious use of social reinforcers. While Goldstein does not discuss his proposals from the same perspective, they are predicated on a symmetrical, equitable relationship between client and therapist, while building personal competence of the clients.

Social attitudes toward the poor, devaluing of the life-style, and refusing to learn and experience the perspective of the poor can indeed preclude effective mental health intervention by the professional. However, this should be understood to result from the mental health worker's own decision not to deal with or confront his prejudices; it is not the inevitable fault of the poor. The change from a condescending, superficial relationship is difficult for most middle-class, upward-striving, mental health professionals. The difficulty is made all the more intractable by the types of training most mental health professionals receive. As exemplified in the Ranz and Dunn chapter, training for working with the poor may require abandoning an entire tradition and may challenge the closely guarded security of many of the current "leaders and directors" of the mental health establishment. Bringing mental health services to the people is a disquieting and unsettling endeavor that does not result in an end product secure and neat—instead the result is a continuing confrontation with real people in real life struggles.

Most mental health professions have been able to continue a relatively platonic existence since their inception, with major professional attention devoted to achieving parity and acceptance with their sister specialties in parent disciplines. Once acceptance is achieved and financial security is assured, there is little incentive for continued reexamination of goals, purposes, or even techniques. Psychiatrists, with their now long-standing tradition of private practice, have the least pressure to concern themselves with care for the poor, though they have successfully competed for leadership roles in community mental health centers. Psychiatric nursing and social work have been much more closely tied to the service of the public through government supported clinics and hospitals. Despite this, the members of these professions have been slow to sense the mental health zeitgeist and to move to meet the apparent needs.

With the development of community mental health centers and the thrust toward providing treatment for all, the mental health professions have made an effort to adapt their skills to the new demands. It has not been enough; the result, in part, has been the development and flourishing of a variety of paraprofessional mental health workers. These individuals have been trained in an array of basic skills and they vary significantly in level of competence as mental health workers. Some are indigenous workers who hopefully can facilitate care in their community of origin. Others have come from outside the community and obtained sub-Bachelor's, or Bachelor's-level degrees in mental health. State governments have moved to create jobs for some of these new roles and in many cases to create career ladders for these new workers. The selection of curricula and amount of training have varied so widely as to be nearly idiosyncratic. The employment of these workers reflects the local needs of the hiring agency far more than the supposed skills obtained by the paraprofessional in training. The result in many cases has been dissatisfied paraprofessionals and further isolation shielding the professions from the consumers—the poor.

Current governmental pressures reflecting the widely held dissatisfaction over financial support of social services for the poor have begun to push for closer accounting of services and for greater participation by the local community in determining the nature and quality of service provided to it.

Mental health programs that were heretofore sacrosanct have been challenged by budget-conscious legislators and administrators and are becoming subject to consumer review. The situation is made even more complex by the intrusion of blatantly political issues into national, statewide, and local funding of mental health programs. Thus, in some cases even programs with adequate justification do not receive continuing support, while others of dubious value receive increased attention. The current zeitgeist makes programs in drug abuse and alcoholism of particular interest, while preventive programs for children go unnoticed and un-funded. "Important" mental health programs come and go, changing to reflect popular public concerns. These changes make it difficult to develop a continuing comprehensive plan of services. Often, as many grant wri-ters can relate, the same program is changed just enough to fit under the guidelines for the latest area of interest in order to maintain funding. Others, no more scrupulous, devise new programs on paper simply to keep the money flowing into the clinic.

Services to the poor seem to have suffered disproportionately in the recent belt tightening because of their lack of political power bases and the prevalent disapproval of "handouts" to the poor. Professionals seek-ing funding for poor-oriented programs often find themselves fighting alone for their own survival without the backing of a strong lobby of consumers. The "poor" consumer has been notably ineffective in creating the national or local demand for mental health services. Riessman pre-dicts that service givers will need to become increasingly consumer con-scious, since consumers will have a major role in the allocation of re-sources. In the case of services to the poor, the consumers will need to be educated and encouraged to actively pursue a consumer advocate role in order to obtain sufficient appropriate service.

The mental health professions will need to respond to their consumers in an open, mutually facilitative way by negotiating with the consumer to adjust and adapt to the changing needs of the community. Those leaders of the professions who have anticipated the changing scene today will have already begun to actively involve the community and to have moved their mental health service business from one of sterile pious immutable status to an open participatory, consumer-oriented service. The mental health worker seeks out his clients and provides the services they want at a time and place suited to the client. Even as consumerism in mental health develops, it is likely that federal policy decisions will have a major impact on the offering of services by virtue of control over the dollar. In order to continue to receive funding, the mental health professions will need to demonstrate their competence and responsiveness to their com-munities. They will require an effective lobby to defeat the opposition of special interests and will have to provide evaluative research and "cost accounting" in order to effectively compete with alternative services for the limited resources. Programs will have to reflect the current attitudes and values of the people.

The value of mental health services to the poor will determine the support and demand for these services. Mental health workers will need to learn to ask for support by "selling" the value of their services to the consumer. The posture of aloof benevolence is likely to lead to termination of funding. To make themselves more efficient, mental health workers will have to specify their goals and target their efforts in order to achieve limited aims. Evaluative research will have an impact on program practice. While decisions of planners and funders are not always predicated on the best research data available, the mental health professions will be well served to lower their resistance to utilizing the findings of good research. As discussed by Shore, research showing effective intervention strategies has been ignored because it is not usefully disseminated, workers are too busy to pay attention, or prejudice prevents acceptance of alternative techniques. As the mental health workers begin to learn about effective and ineffective strategies, research learnings should be utilized in the expanding and offering of new services. We can ill afford continuing to ignore evaluative program research in the increasingly competitive marketplace of services.

Traditional therapy (as a tertiary treatment) will probably diminish in importance in the coming decades. Schlesinger argues that it is too inefficient to survive the increasing pressure for service to people in trouble. One of the ways in which primary and secondary prevention strategies will be enhanced is through the development of inter- and intraagency linkages. One of the increasingly apparent difficulties in solving any personal problems is in finding and coordinating services and institutional responses to the individual. Progress in the area of social institution integration, linkage, and coordination could have a major impact on the mental health services. For the first time, this could permit the mental health worker to deal, in ombudsman fashion, with the myriad of reality problems that have exacerbated the psychopathological symptomatology of the client, especially the socioeconomically poor client. Little concerted work has been done in this area but, as evidenced by some current federally sponsored research, a systematic effort is now underway to determine the social service linkages, to measure their impact, and to find ways to alter them. These are monumental tasks but deserve the energies of the most creative among us.

A part of the mental health worker's adjustment to the needs of the poor lies in social action. Reiff makes a strong argument that much social action has been ill thought out and ultimately works to the continuing detriment of the people it was designed to help. Wolpe has shown that major changes can be wrought, in Nader fashion, from head-on assault on inequities. She also demonstrates that one sensitive mental health worker can have a major impact in a social crisis of substantial proportion. So, with the Reiff caveat, it seems evident that many of the problems that receive continuing worry and concern could be appreciably and materially influenced by direct, concerted effort. False crusades, however, can be of harm to those they are supposed to save, leaving the mental health professional relatively unscathed. The decision to undertake dramatic Alinsky-type social action strategies requires serious conceptual and participating involvement, consideration of the ethical and value questions, and an analysis of the possible consequences to the client population.

The reader of this volume is likely to be in a position to act on behalf of the mental health interests of the poor. While each of the chapter authors has made his point, it will take the direct action of others to have these points result in important change. Here we cite five general recommendations applicable to a range of mental health concerns.

1. Each of the authors represented in this book has demonstrated at least one thing in common. Each is actively involved in mental health services to the poor. While the contributions have covered the range from theoretical to practical, all have invested themselves heavily in the endeavor. All have gone beyond criticism to conceptualize, propose, and implement action alternatives. Changes in the delivery of service to the poor will come about only to the degree that individuals work for that change. We each have the potential for action and the responsibility for action on one or more fronts. Opportunities for work abound at all levels, and include the political arena, our professional guilds, manpower training programs, and direct service work.

2. In the process of deciding what actions to take, it is essential to analyze our conceptual system, including the subtle and indirect prejudgments that determine the models underlying our actions. Personal change on a broad scale may require the ability to consider alternative conceptions of reality. As a consequence of these analyses, it should be possible to produce an honest confrontation of our own motives and the implicit goals of the professional associations to which we belong. The seemingly benevolent policies of the mental health establishment can be used to justify the continuation of policies that ignore the mental health problems of the poor.

3. The ideal mental health service, for the poor or others, should have clearly specified goals and should be answerable to those goals. The designers and implementers of mental health programs should know

the goals of the programs and should be prepared to adjust their work to meet these goals. The use of specifiable goals will permit the evaluation of the program; they can be used to indicate the directions for improvement and to help in the search for continued financial and administrative support. The evaluation strategy should endeavor to obtain enough measures involving differing methods so that the goal construct can be fairly assessed. Social, zeitgeist, or psychological goals are legitimate and may be of overriding importance. It is often necessary to justify the program in terms of these currently popular beliefs and values.

4. The nature of service to the urban poor should enhance the competence of the consumer. Services should not seek to create a client in the image of the middle class, but should build on the unique skills of the recipient and be consistent with his values. This requires individual assessment of the consumer and his needs, and it implies that programs should be developed with full consumer input and participation. The services should be integrated. Effective coordination and utilization of a variety of resources multiplies the impact of one individual and, given the pervasive nature of many problems, offers one reasonable strategy for effective mastery. Integration and coordination produce the opportunity to build coalitions made up of disparate groups with often conflicting motives united on the cause in question.

5. Finally, it is important that workers in mental health be fully cognizant of the impact of their actions on the consumer and the community, especially important in major social action strategies. Attention to values and the impact of programs on human relationships, personal feelings, and individual competence is essential for the ethical worker.

In some ways we have seen that the mental health problems of the urban poor are isomorphic with the mental health problems of us all; insofar as this is true, strategies of effective intervention are basically the same. Some of the unique aspects of the urban poor that indicate adjustment in approach have been highlighted in this book in ways that should provoke thought and stimulate action.

It is becoming increasingly clear that no single model will encompass all of the concerns, issues, or perspectives relating to mental health and the poor. Each of the models represented by the chapters presented in this book contribute unique views with particular consequences. In some cases the logical consequences of the differing models conflict in emphasis or substance. As a result, the reader is left to review and balance the insights provided against the reality of his experience. These chapters should help the process of developing our understanding and appreciation of the problems in implementing a strategy of mental health services for the urban poor.

REFERENCE

Goldstein, A. *Structured learning therapy: Toward a psychotherapy for the poor.* New York: Academic Press, 1973.

Index

TITLES IN THE PERGAMON GENERAL PSYCHOLOGY SERIES